"I thoroughly enjoyed reading this very important and heartfelt book about allergies in children. Uche's personal journey managing her lovely daughter's allergies to the point that she is allergy-free and thriving, is refreshing to read and offers a ray of hope to all in the same boat.

I would recommend this book to all parents and carers of children with allergies, as well as all clinicians who are in contact with children."

DR. ADAEZE IFEZULIKE, MBE

Primary Care and Lifestyle Medicine Physician

"Uche's book is a narrative of her personal journey managing her daughter's allergies which, together with her scientific background and knowledge and an incredible willingness to learn and understand, is a winning combination to imparting both knowledge and wisdom. I am so grateful that Uche has taken the time and effort to write this important book. It will be a helpful read to all parents and carers who find themselves on any leg of this journey with allergies."

NICOLA MCCLEAN

Specialist Paediatric Dietitian

"I like the way you personalise it [the book]. I also really like the take-home messages which are good key points of learning. It is an excellent, clear and easy read. This book will increase people's knowledge and provide a calm and confidence to families. Well done! I will be intrigued if you write another book a few years down the line."

ALICE HOLMES

Lead Clinical Nurse for Cambridge Children's Hospital

"I have read your story and it is very moving. Very well done for taking on such a task in addressing your daughter's allergies for the longer-term benefit, and succeeding at it too. Well done, Uche. This is a book that will help so many people as the incidence of allergy is rising."

CORA MCKEOWN

Patient, Public & Professional Experience Manager
New Hospitals Programme, NHS England

THRIVE
ALLERGY FREE

Journey to a life unlimited by food allergies

DR. UCHE OKORJI-OBIKE

THRIVE ALLERGY FREE

Editing by Rhoda Molife

Inner Layout & Cover Design by Aqua Media & Publishing (AMP) Studios (aquapubng@gmail.com)

DEDICATION

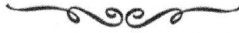

To my miracle daughter, Chimamanda - your mighty resilience inspired me to write this book so that our story can inspire someone else to thrive allergy free.

ACKNOWLEDGEMENTS

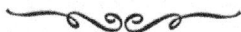

To my sunshine, Chimamanda Michelle – it's a pleasure being your mummy every day. You are such a joy and just beautiful inside and out. Your gorgeous smile and your mighty resolve, even when your eczema and allergies were at their worst, have given me the drive to complete this book. You may not know it yet but our journey has taught me a lot about parenting and helped me to positively impact the lives of others. I hope one day you will see how many lives you have blessed and inspired.

To my precious gem of a husband, Nnamdi - thank you for always being there. Thanks for your encouragement and being my consistent cheerleader in all that I do, especially when writing this book.

I also have such an appreciation for my family – my parents, siblings, mother-in-law, sisters- and brothers-in-law, who are forever supportive of me and Nnamdi. A special thanks to my mum who spent nearly three months with us after Chimamanda was born supporting us in every way possible. Mums are superheroes!

To my friends and church family - thanks for checking on and supporting us throughout the journey with Chimamanda. Thanks for always readily accommodating her food allergies.

To the healthcare professionals who have worked with us from diagnosis through reintroduction and to recovery, you are all superstars. We could not have gotten here without you all. A special thanks to our dermatology nurse and Nicola McLean, our paediatric dietitian, both of whom made the journey not just manageable but also memorable.

To the reviewers, thanks a lot for gifting me with your precious time to go through this book and sharing your honest thoughts on the work. I really appreciate your comments and recommended resources that have added to the depth of this book.

Special thanks to my editor Rhoda Molife for all her contributions towards whipping this book into shape. I am glad I worked with you on this project.

TABLE OF CONTENTS

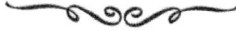

FOREWORD BY

AllergyUK

*R*eceiving a diagnosis of a food allergy can be a daunting and overwhelming experience, particularly for parents with a young child who may already be overwhelmed by parenthood.

Uche provides an honest account of the diagnosis and management of food allergy in her little girl, Chimamanda. Her book also weaves in the most up-to-date scientific information in an easy-to-understand and digestible way. She reflects on all aspects of Chimamanda's condition and care including her eczema, allergy testing, how she dealt with reintroduction, as well as the importance of getting timely advice from specialists in the field. The account not only offers practical support for children with food allergy but also helps to reduce parental anxiety and reinforces the importance of self-care.

Lived experiences of others are a valuable way of building knowledge around how to manage food allergies. Diverse representation in the voice of this lived experience is vital for conveying how allergy does not discriminate; it really can affect anyone of us.

Uche recognises that as someone of African heritage and with a scientific background, her journey is a unique addition to the conversation around allergy.

I have no doubt that this book will help those in the allergic community who are feeling lost and seeking reassurance from someone who has gone from diagnosis right through to resolution.

LYDIA COLLINS-HUSSEY
Clinical Dietetic Advisor
Allergy UK

PREFACE

> *Knowledge is power, Information is liberating. Education is the premise of progress, in every society, in every family.* – Kofi Annan

First, let me say that I am super thrilled that you picked up this book. By doing this, you have taken an important step to understanding and overcoming the challenges that come with food allergies.

Three months after my daughter was born, she was diagnosed with cow's milk protein allergy (CMPA) and egg allergy. It turned out to be a defining time for us as a family. Along the way, I developed this urge to help others who were going through what we were and enlighten those who wanted to learn more about food allergies. I had always been a private person, so to share this was going to be a huge challenge for me. What drove me though was the realisation that opening up and sharing my experiences and knowledge had not only been helpful for my husband and I but also for others. Many who were going through similar experiences and unsure of what to do, gravitated towards me. Through our discussions, they learnt so much, so I had to continue the work.

Now, there are three 'es' in learning: education, exposure and experience. My research doctorate - education - and work investigates inflammation (which is the mechanism behind allergic responses and many other diseases). Being exposed to the effects then brings a greater depth to the knowledge I gained. However, it is a completely different ball game when you have a lived experience. To witness the manifestation of science in live and living colour with my little one was an experience like no other. So, through my work and family's journey, I lived these three modes of learning and I strongly felt that what I came to know could help someone.

The first idea that came to mind was to create an online resource for parents and families of children with allergies. So, in September 2021 I launched Tots2Teens Allergies which is an allergy communication service and consultancy that gives professional information and recommends services for parents and carers of children with allergies. Writing a book about our family experience is complementary to the platform as our story was the inspiration behind Tots2Teens Allergies.

I hope this book becomes a useful 'go-to guide' on your journey to understanding and living with food allergies; a guide that can help transition you to effortless living with allergies. It may also be useful for the extended family, friends, teachers and carers of those with allergies as well as those who just want to learn more about the condition.

Together, we can thrive, allergy free.

INTRODUCTION

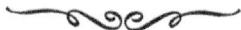

*T*his book is for you, yes you:

- a parent of a child with food allergies

- someone who wants to learn about food allergies

- someone who wants to support those with allergies

- a childcare professional who works with babies, toddlers and children who are exploring food

- a teacher, carer or healthcare professional who works with children and wants to learn more about their food allergies

Let's start with some statistics. Did you know that:

- 3 – 6% of children in the developed world have a food allergy[1].

- In western countries, challenge-diagnosed food allergy was reported to be as high as 10%[2].

- In the United Kingdom (UK), 6 - 8% of children up to the age of three have a food allergy[3].

- A UK study reported the prevalence of food allergy as 7.1% in breast-fed infants[1],[4].

- Children with early-onset eczema have a higher risk of developing food allergy[5,6].

- Egg allergy, cow's milk protein allergy (CMPA) and peanut allergy are the most common food allergies in children[7].

- According to the Breastfeeding Network UK, between 2% and 7.5% of formula-fed and 0.5% of exclusively breast-fed babies develop CMPA[8].

- 1 in 5 children develop a peanut allergy by the age of five[9].

- In the United States (US), it is estimated that peanut allergy affects 0.8% of children whilst in the UK around 2% of children are affected[9]. Another study reported the prevalence of peanut allergy to be 1.34% in a Canadian province amongst primary school children[10]. In Australia, 3% of children aged one year have a peanut allergy[11].

- The prevalence of CMPA in children aged 0 to 5 years is 2%[12].

- About 50% of children with CMPA suffer from eczema and gastrointestinal symptoms[13,14].

- In the US, a survey revealed a prevalence of 8% for food allergy in children less than 18 years old[2].

- In Latin America, a review of data suggested that sensitization to peanuts is low. However, there was a high frequency of sensitisation to fish and fruits and most of the data suggested food allergies were predominant in children under the age of five[15]

- The evidence shows a rise in the prevalence of food allergy in developing countries, with rates of diagnosed food allergy in Africa reported to be similar to that reported in Western countries[2].

- A study by Kung *et al* reviewing studies in Ghana, Nigeria, Kenya, Tanzania, Mozambique, Botswana and South Africa, suggested that there was an increase in food allergy in those countries. This highlights that food allergy is an emerging problem on the African continent[16].

- Kung *et al*'s review found that 26% of oral food challenge-proven peanut allergy was observed in patients with eczema in South Africa. In addition, a study conducted in south-eastern Nigeria showed that 4% of the population studied with allergies to eggs, crayfish and milk, also had eczema.

- Interestingly, it has been observed that children of East Asian or African descent born in western environments are at higher risk of food allergy compared to Caucasian children[2].

- According to Food Allergy Research and Education (FARE) about 40% of children with food allergies are allergic to more than one food[17].

- Worldwide, 1 in 8 children have asthma and 1 in 8 children have allergic rhinitis.

- It has been reported that sensitivity to food is more frequent in people with allergic diseases such as asthma and eczema. Today, it is well documented that the strongest risk factor for food allergies is eczema, especially eczema that starts early in life and which is more severe[18].

There you go. These are the statistics and the numbers show that food allergy is a very important condition.

Some might ask why this is the case. There are different hypotheses out there. In a presentation at the Joint World Allergy Organisation (WAO) and British Society for Allergy and Clinical Immunology (BSACI) conference in April 2022, Hugh Sampson summarised the key causes:

- changes in the environment due to a modern lifestyle, industrialisation and urbanisation

- increased prevalence of eczema

Interestingly, race and ethnic disparities in western countries have been implicated, as studies have shown that people of colour have higher rates of food allergies.

The question then is, what has been done with these statistics? The answer? Quite a lot. Healthcare professionals have established sound diagnosis and management plans for children with allergies. Scientists continue to research the causes and apply cutting edge technology to develop effective treatments. But what can we do? Well, parents of children with food allergies have access to the same information that healthcare professionals and scientists have, and they can use this knowledge to best care for their child with allergies.

Others – teachers, relatives, friends and carers - can do the same to help them support these children in their care. New or expecting parents can be on guard for food allergies and use what others know to their advantage.

So, what is thriving allergy free? Can one become allergy free? The answer is, 'yes, they can'. In this book, thriving allergy free is:

- having the right management plan in place so that children and their parents do not live in fear of an allergic reaction

- having the right resources to enable one to live a fulfilled life with allergies

- living a life unlimited by food allergies

- a successful reintroduction of a trigger food

My daughter was diagnosed with food allergies as a baby and has gone on to thrive, allergy free. As you go through the pages of this book, you will learn more about her journey. In addition, if you are not already aware of her, look up Shiv Sewlal. She is an allergy advocate who I first came across on the FARE social media platforms. Shiv was born with 40-plus food allergies as well as eczema. That is all she has ever known, and she is living life to the fullest whilst creating awareness.

Through the course of researching and writing this book, I met families whose children live with food allergies; some were not aware that they could reintroduce their children to the trigger food, whilst others feared the idea. There were others who reintroduced foods successfully, working with healthcare professionals. I also met parents who took matters into their own hands and found their own solutions which were not necessarily appropriate.

You will see that I throw in some science and medical terms. Do not be intimidated by this. We are all the embodiment of science which means science is for all of us. I will break down any complex concepts though, as well as direct you to additional resources to expand your knowledge and increase your confidence. These extra resources can be printed out and kept as posters or cards for easy reference. Finally, at the end of each chapter will be a summary of the take-home messages that you can refer to at any time.

So, let's go and learn about how to thrive allergy free!

Chapter One

IS YOUR BABY A BOY OR A GIRL?

'No one else will ever know the strength of my love for you. After all, you're the only one who knows what my heart sounds like from the inside.' – Unknown

Giving birth to my daughter, Chimamanda, in 2019 was one of the most beautiful things I had ever experienced and one of the best things that has ever happened to me. The sheer joy of looking at my baby and the amazement that this little person was birthed by me was mind-blowing. A mini-me! Above all, I rejoiced and remain very grateful for the miracle of conception, the grace to carry the pregnancy to term and the joy that comes with delivery. Becoming a mum changes a person; no matter how different our experiences, it makes us better people who learn how to truly care and love wholeheartedly. I hope that every parent and soon-to-be mum or dad going through the pages of this book gets to a stage where they treasure the beauty of it all and appreciate this great miracle.

As a first-time mum, I soaked up the experience and dwelt in every moment of loving my baby girl. My husband and I were looking forward to the adventure of parenting. Though we had no idea of what the future held, we did not expect that we were going to be raising a child with severe eczema and food allergies.

Following Chimamanda's birth, it soon became apparent that she was not latching well during breastfeeding. She was also very clingy and easily irritable. After many discussions, our health visitor suggested a nipple cap, so we invested in a range of these. They did not help. We were subsequently seen by another health visitor who suggested a meeting with a lactation consultant. We saw one who confirmed that Chimamanda was not latching well because she had a tongue-tie. Good – we had found the problem that had a solution.

Whilst we were waiting for Chimamanda to undergo division of the tongue-tie, I was expressing breast milk for bottle-feeding whilst encouraging her to latch and breastfeed as much as she could. All of this was not part of my plan which was to exclusively breastfeed at least for six months and without bottles. Fortunately, the division was done by the time she was one month old. Things improved dramatically and I thought, *Great, we're back on track.* However, my gorgeous girl remained clingy.

In between all this, I had also noticed that some of the spots on her skin which she had at birth were not going away and her skin was getting drier by the day.

This really did not matter too much until it came to her first baby photoshoot. It had been booked well in advance and had to be done as soon as possible after birth, when she was still very flexible and able to maintain the foetal position for a good stretch of time. It should have been a joyous experience but it was far from that. Chimamanda was cranky throughout and we had no idea that her skin was being irritated by the repeated outfit changes. Our photographer was ever so gentle and kind though, but this, in hindsight, was a sign that all was not well with our child.

Over the following months, Chimamanda's clinginess got worse, her skin became drier and drier, and she started staying on longer during breastfeeding just to soothe herself. Mind you, whilst I was pregnant, we had carried out a deep clean of the house as we were mindful that dust mites and environmental *triggers* could cause several reactions. So we were a bit flummoxed; surely, we had done everything possible to protect her. Consultations with the health visitors and our general practitioner (GP; family doctor) gave no obvious cause for her discontent and dry skin. My husband, Nnamdi, a medical doctor himself who also had experience in paediatrics, thought it was eczema as this is quite common in children; we decided to run with that. We tried different baby lotions, potions and even homemade recipes using oils like coconut and olive oil as well as shea butter. None of these helped. Our GP gave prescribed treatments which also did nothing.

It got to the stage where Chimamanda had to be cuddled to sleep because she was so irritable. At our baby groups, I was in awe of babies who slept on their own and throughout the night because that was not my experience at all. Thankfully, we had my mother. She had started living with us when Chimamanda was a week old and took it upon herself to spend the nights with her. This meant I could sleep in between feeds, especially when my husband had finished his two-week paternity leave.

As her skin worsened, we suspected that she had an allergy though we had no idea what the trigger was. She drank breast milk and nothing else, and we made sure that her skin came into contact with cotton material only. We even put her woollen outfits on top of her cotton ones so that at least she could get some wear out of the many gifts she had. As far as we could tell, we were doing everything possible to protect her skin, yet nothing seemed to work. Before we knew it, she developed severe cradle cap and her hair fell out with each stroke of a comb. Everything was changing so fast and I, the mum-scientist, and my husband the dad-doctor, had run out of ideas. We knew we needed to do more.

One day we woke up and Chimamanda's hair was gone. All that remained were a few strands on her eyebrows. When we were out and about, people who walked up to take a closer look at her would ask, "Is your baby a boy or girl?" At first, I would answer without a second thought, but soon it became annoying. Even though I knew that sometimes it was difficult to tell the gender difference in babies, surely even without hair, one could tell that Chimamanda was a girl. Then it dawned on me that normally baby girls would wear a headband or ribbon. My baby could not. I did not dare accessorise her outfits with anything else but the bare minimum in case her skin reacted. The other thing was that I had only bought gender neutral outfits for her. However, after being repeatedly asked 'the question', one day I bought an entire wardrobe of pink outfits to provide the answer before I was asked. That did not help entirely as some still said, "Oh *he*'s so gorgeous."

Next Chimamanda's skin became scaly and cracked. We were still consulting the GP regularly, trying new prescriptions and getting more frustrated. Mothers at our baby groups offered many suggestions including cleaning her skin with breast milk. I had gotten to the stage where I would try anything because by then, quite frankly, her skin looked like that of a reptile. The turning point came when it started to crack then developed open sores that became infected. I asked our GP to refer her to a consultant *paediatric dermatologist* and she was started on antibiotics in the meantime. This was a picture I or no parent wanted to see: their child suffering, helpless and unable to communicate how he or she was feeling. The tortuous part was the feeling of inadequacy as neither of us had been able to help her. As we waited for the *dermatology* appointment, it was now clear to us that there was something serious going on. And to make it more challenging, by this time, my mother had finished her three-month stint with us and so it was left to Nnamdi and I to carry on.

Alongside the eczema, what we had noticed was that Chimamanda was not gaining weight at all. People would often pass comments on how small she was. "Oh, she's a tiny baby" or "Tiny, tiny baby", were frequent passing comments. This infuriated me more than the gender question, especially as weight is such a focus in those first few months of a baby's life. If a child is not gaining weight, it makes one feel particularly inadequate. I know most parents can identify with this feeling - that you are not feeding your child enough. I later discovered, in my many conversations with parents of children with food allergies, that weight gain or rather the lack of it was a major concern too. We were so desperate to help Chimamanda that whilst we waited for her appointment, we introduced a bit of formula to help her gain weight. In hindsight that was a bad move as her skin flared up more.

The day of the appointment finally arrived, just a few days before Christmas 2019. When we arrived at the clinic in Addenbrookes Hospital, Cambridge (UK), we first saw Karen Tabor, a lovely consultant dermatology nurse. She examined Chimamanda so gently. Following her examination, she went on to discuss things with the consultant dermatologist. On her return, she explained that Chimamanda would have an allergy test and a new treatment plan for her skin care. I felt a mixture of anxiety and relief - anxiety that there may be something seriously wrong with my daughter's health and relief that maybe we were coming to the end of whatever it was. Though we by now suspected that she had an allergy,

I remained hopeful that this was not the case. We were more reassured than we had been in a long time that was for sure.

The result of the allergy test came back on Christmas Eve and was positive for CMPA and egg allergy. This was not a Christmas present I was expecting. Even more complicated was that apparently, she was reacting to the milk and egg protein in my diet. This was unusual as most food allergy stems from ingesting the trigger. The other potential culprit was the formula milk we had just added to her diet. We were immediately referred to a paediatric dietitian, Nicola McLean, for follow up and it was recommended that for the time being I had to stop eating food containing egg and cow's milk should I want to continue breastfeeding. A *hypoallergenic* milk formula was also prescribed. No more stabbing in the dark - we were now hitting the target. This was a step in the right direction as we embarked on our journey to recovery.

My scientific curiosity went up a gear. I needed to understand what was happening to my daughter and what I could do to help her, even with the close guidance we were now getting. I read scientific articles, books and any kind of literature that could teach me more about food allergy. Having researched the field of inflammation for a long time, I invested in understanding how what I knew translated to real life. I also joined the British Society for Allergy and Clinical Immunology (BSACI) and attended a lot of their webinars, grand rounds (where they discuss real patient cases) and lectures. I am excited to share some of what

I learnt with you in the upcoming chapters.

Two important things I learnt during this period were that:

- food allergy is complex

- healthcare professionals take making the correct diagnosis seriously

It sometimes felt that our GP was not moving fast enough towards a diagnosis for Chimamanda. However, in hindsight and despite the frustrations, they had to follow due process and did their job to the best of their ability. One piece of advice I will share with you, even if you do not have a scientific or medical background, is not to hesitate to ask for what you think is best for your child. For us, it was one thing to have the knowledge but another to live the experience. We lived it. So, be guided by what you are living and if that is uncomfortable, seek and ask for what you and your child need to make things comfortable.

Take Home Messages

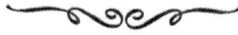

- Life can throw you a curveball at any time. How do you catch that ball and what do you do with it? Roll it about in our hands? Squeeze it? Bounce it? For me, I did all three to find out what I could do. I read, researched and learnt again. You, by reading this book, are doing the same. Well done and continue your quest.

- It is important to seek the help of healthcare professionals. Even with our science backgrounds, Nnamdi and I did not try to work things out alone and we followed independent medical guidance. Getting to a diagnosis is like completing a puzzle; different pieces (of information) must be put together. Sometimes the pieces need to be moved around so more hands working together usually mean the puzzle is solved faster. For an accurate diagnosis and effective treatment plan, ask for and accept help.

Chapter Two

ECZEMA AND FOOD ALLERGY

"Caring for a child with an allergy can feel like a lonely journey but remember that you are not alone." – Uche Okorji-Obike

What is Eczema?

Eczema is a term that refers to a group of conditions that causes *inflammation* of the skin making it discoloured and itchy. This group of conditions are generally referred to as *dermatitis*. There are different types of eczema that are common in children and include:

1. *atopic dermatitis* - the skin is itchy, dry and cracked and most often found in those with allergies or who have family members affected by eczema, asthma or hay fever

2. *contact dermatitis* - eczema triggered by contact with a particular substance

3. *dyshidrotic eczema* - eczema that affects the hands or feet. It is also known as pompholyx

4. *seborrheic dermatitis* – commonly known as *cradle cap* and refers to eczema that appears where there are a lot of oil-producing glands like the back, nose, and scalp

In the rest of the book, when I say eczema, I will be referring primarily to atopic dermatitis unless otherwise stated.

Eczema is different in everyone. In my conversations with parents of children with black and brown skin, there were always concerns that the appearance of skin conditions, not just eczema, in different skin tones was not at all well appreciated by healthcare professionals. The typical description for eczema refers to 'red' skin. Well, black and brown skins do not become red but white skin does. I have a dark skin tone and so does my daughter and neither of us have ever had redness. It would not be surprising if this limited understanding results in delayed diagnosis, and it certainly highlights an important gap in knowledge and medical care. In my research, I was pleased to come across work that is trying to fill this gap. A medical student in London, Malone Mukwende, co-wrote a clinical handbook of images of skin conditions in black and brown skins called *Mind the Gap*. He wrote this book after he realised that none of his clinical tutors could tell him how skin conditions would manifest in black and brown skin. The resource has had a global impact on inclusivity and the quality of medical education and health care. Malone has gone on to create a resource, *Hutano*, a social health platform for black and brown people to discuss all aspects of their health www.tryhutano.com. In recent times, we are beginning to see a new breed of medics and medics-in-training who are speaking up on the need for diversity and representation in all aspects of medicine especially for black and brown skin - a step in the right direction for all.

FOOD ALLERGY AND ECZEMA: IS THERE A CONNECTION?

It is widely thought that eczema is the result of food allergy. You may also know that many people with eczema can have hay fever and asthma. What is clear is that these conditions are all linked to the immune system. More on the immune system in the next chapter.

A study carried out by the Murdoch Children's Research Institute in Australia reported that 1 in 5 infants with eczema were allergic to peanut, egg white or sesame compared to 1 in 25 infants without eczema. The same study also found that infants with eczema were 11 times more likely to develop a peanut allergy and approximately 6% more likely to develop egg allergy by the age of one than infants without eczema. Finally, their results showed that about 50% of infants with early onset eczema (that started at less than 3 months old) who were treated with topical corticosteroid (a type of steroid applied to the skin) developed food allergy. In another study in Europe, it was found that the worse eczema was, the higher the chance of developing an egg allergy. What these pieces of research (and others too) show is that there is a link between eczema and food allergy, but it is not so clear cut.

––––––––––––––––

"Not every baby with eczema has a food allergy (and vice versa), but the earlier the onset and the more severe the eczema is, the more likely it is to be associated with a food allergy."

~ Paula Hallam, Paediatric Dietitian

––––––––––––––––

THE TRIGGERS

At birth, babies are all at risk of developing eczema. Research suggests that this is related to a combination of genetic and environmental factors. There are certain *genes* that if abnormal can increase the risk of developing eczema. Environmental substances – the *triggers* – can further disrupt the skin and this may cause eczema. The extent of the abnormality in any one gene or set of genes or the combination of genes and environmental factors that interplay can vary between individuals. This makes it difficult to predict who will get eczema and how severe it will be. Whilst we cannot alter these genes, we can identify the triggers, and this may either prevent eczema or minimise the severity.

The triggers for eczema in babies range from toiletries to foods. Some of the most common ones in babies include heat, soap, fabrics especially wool, house dust mites, pollen, animal dander and viral or bacterial infections. Once a trigger has been identified, it is important to remove it and avoid it.

ABOUT THE SKIN OF BABES

In my conversations with a dermatologist I had connected with, Dr Folakemi Cole-Adeife, I learnt that the neonatal skin care routine in the first few days of life was very important in maintaining a baby's skin health and minimising the risk of eczema. She mentioned something that struck me – in western Nigeria, there is a tradition of washing a new baby in palm oil to create a protective layer on the skin. There are probably similar practices around the globe too and I think that the idea behind this is to lock moisture in the child's skin.

The development of a baby's protective skin barrier starts at the time of the vaginal birth when the baby is exposed to various components of the maternal *microbe*. This maternal-infant microbial transfer helps equip the baby's skin for the world. Within a few weeks of birth, the skin changes from a neutral to an *acidic pH*. This acidic film on the surface of the skin is called the *acid mantle* and is a protective barrier. Where the water is soft and therefore acidic like the acid mantle, a water-only bath works best. Where the water is hard and *alkaline*, a water only bath may disturb the acid mantle causing dry skin. Here, a mild liquid baby cleanser or sensitive fragrance-free wipes may work better.

A significant disruption to the formation of this protective barrier can lead to impaired skin function which makes it vulnerable to chemical damage, infections and other skin diseases. Premature babies are particularly at risk, and if you have seen one, you can see that their skin is yet to mature fully. Here, adequate skin care is crucial. Studies have also shown that having a *Caesarean delivery* (C-section) eliminates that opportunity for the maternal-infant microbial transfer and so can increase the subsequent risk for eczema. However, there is a conflict of opinions between experts on the relationship between the development of eczema and C-section.

A recent study carried out by Professor Carsten Flohr of the St John's Institute of Dermatology King's College and published in 2019, showed a link between gut bacteria and infant diet, eczema and C-section. The study known as Enquiring About Tolerance (EAT), showed that babies born by C-section had a less diverse *gut flora*, compared to those delivered by vaginal birth. It was also shown that babies who had eczema at three months and one year of age showed a higher abundance of a particular type of bacteria called *Clostridium sensu stricto* when compared to those without eczema. These results suggested that there is an important relationship between the type of bacteria in the gut and the development of eczema and food allergies early in life.

*"The British Skin Foundation is delighted to have funded [this]
research [study] into the role of the gut microbiome in the
development of eczema and food allergies in early life. Since there
seems to be a relationship between the type of bacteria in the gut
and the development of eczema, the manipulation of the gut
bacteria in early life might reduce the likelihood of eczema in
babies predisposed to developing it."*

~ Professor David Gawkrodger, British Skin Foundation Trustee
and Consultant Dermatologist

So, what can be done for those babies with a higher
risk of developing eczema? Encouraging a diverse
microbiome is essential in helping a child develop their
immune system. *Probiotics*, known as 'friendly' live
bacteria, and yeasts which are usually added to
yoghurts, can do this. They are thought to be beneficial
because they help restore the natural balance of
bacteria in the gut. *Prebiotics* are a group of some plant
fibres that these 'friendly' gut bacteria feed which also
help in diversifying the gut microbiome. Most
importantly, input from a dietitian is important. In
addition to increasing the gut microbiome, the EAT
study suggested that early introduction of *allergenic*
foods accelerated the development of greater gut
bacteria diversity when compared to exclusive
breastfeeding.

PRINCIPLES OF SKIN CARE

When it comes to taking care of a baby's skin, little or nothing is generally required. It is important to avoid chemicals, fragrances and dyes in clothing. If excessively dry skin develops, the first step here is always to identify the cause which is the crux to making a diagnosis, then avoiding it. You may also need a healthcare professional to help with this and of course with treatment.

Here is a summary of the treatments that are likely to be offered to you. One of the most important things is to keep the skin moisturised and protected and emollients are used to do this. Emollients are moisturisers that soothe and hydrate the skin. There are four types:

LOTION - these are thin emollients that can spread easily and so are suitable for hairy or damaged skin areas that are weeping. They are easily absorbed and are great in hot weather.

CREAM - creams are slightly thicker than lotions, not so greasy and are quickly absorbed. They can be substitutes for soap since soap can dry out the skin, something to avoid with severe eczema.

GEL - Gels are thick emollients, thicker than lotions. They work best if you need something that has a long-lasting effect.

OINTMENT - These are the thickest of the emollients, are oily and so feel very greasy. They are great for very dry skin as they are super moisturising.

Being free from preservatives makes them good for sensitive skin. An ointment worked best for my daughter; in my conversations, I found a lot of black people felt an ointment worked best for their skin type.

Generally, the thin emollients like lotions and creams are easily absorbed but will require frequent application. The thicker gels and ointments are needed for severe dryness and require less reapplication. To find out more about the different emollients explore the resources available at the following website: www.tots2teensallergies.com/thrive.

If skin flare ups, rashes, excessive itching and redness – all signs of inflammation - appear, then topical corticosteroids may be prescribed. These steroids are anti-inflammatory which means they reduce inflammation. When the skin is itchy, naturally your child will want to scratch but this increases the risk of breaking the skin barrier leading to infection. Whilst you can encourage them not to scratch, it is easier said than done and so the use of emollients and topical steroids when needed are important.

One thing I found useful were wet wraps. They worked wonders in rehydrating and calming the skin and appeared to make the topical treatments more effective. A wet wrap is a wet dressing used to rehydrate the skin. You can make one easily yourself with a gauze or cotton fabric which is dampened with warm water and then applied to affected areas after using an emollient; they work best after a bath and after applying a topical medication and/or emollient. The wrap can then be left for a few hours or overnight.

Common brands that make wearable material for wet wraps are Skinnies® and Comfifast® garments. More information on eczema and skin care is available at www.tots2teensallergies.com/thrive

Take Home Messages

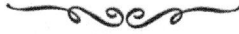

- Eczema is linked to food allergies but not all cases of eczema are associated with or lead to food allergy.

- Research suggests that there is a link between the gut microbiome, eczema and food allergies.

- The diagnosis of eczema should always be made by a doctor. Online kits for allergy testing without proper guidance and interpretation of results is not recommended.

- Probiotics and prebiotics can stimulate the expansion of a diverse microbiome in your child.

- Effective skin care for children with eczema is based around keeping the skin moisturised with emollients.

Chapter Three

UNDERSTANDING FOOD HYPERSENSITIVITY, FOOD ALLERGY AND FOOD INTOLERANCE

"Unless we learn to know ourselves, we run the danger of destroying ourselves." – Ja A Jahannes

$\mathscr{A}$s a scientist, food allergy, food sensitivity and allergic reactions were phrases that I was very much aware of. However, I had no idea how much of a personal meaning these words would come to hold for me. Most people refer to food allergy with little or no understanding of what it means, and this may contribute to the seemingly rising number of children with food allergies. Many of these cases are not actually confirmed. In fact, the term 'overdiagnosis of allergy' has been coined by doctors to describe the phenomenon where many parents and carers conclude that their little ones have an allergy to a particular food that has not been medically diagnosed.

Children by and large get to know who they are through their parents and carers, so it is important for parents to equip themselves with the right knowledge to allow them to teach their children. So, let us clarify what *food hypersensitivity*, *food allergy* and *food intolerance* are, but first, a little fun with science.

THE IMMUNE SYSTEM AND ALLERGIC REACTIONS

The *immune system* is a network of cells, organs, proteins known as *antibodies* and chemicals that together function as a safety surveillance system for the body. It is always on the lookout for harmful foreign substances such as bacteria and viruses as well as our own cells that may 'go bad'. When the system comes across such a situation, it sets off the antibodies to find, latch on to and kick start the process of destroying the harmful substance. Various chemicals are released in this process; this usually all happens without us really knowing or feeling anything. Sometimes the immune system goes into overdrive and mistakenly identifies something as harmful when it really is not. This 'something' is called an *allergen*. When the immune system reacts to an allergen, the immediate response is the release of a particular type of antibody known as *IgE* and chemicals known as *histamines*. Histamines make blood vessels expand, releasing other chemicals that cause what we see as an allergic reaction.

Therefore, *antihistamines* are used to treat an allergic reaction as these drugs counteract the main cause of the allergic reaction – histamines.

In delayed reactions, the process is different. What is called a *cell-mediated* reaction occurs and it is not as well understood as the immediate reaction. Another group of cells known as T-cells are involved (they are also triggered in immediate reactions described above too). *Cytokines* are small proteins which create signals that lead to a delayed reaction. These processes can happen with any allergy, including food allergy. A pictorial illustration can be downloaded from www.tots2teensallergies.com/thrive

A LITTLE MORE ON ALLERGENS

An allergen is the cause of an allergic reaction. I will also refer to it as a trigger. Only small amounts of an allergen are needed to cause a reaction. The most common allergens are:

- animal proteins like that found in house dust mites
- pollen
- venom in insect bites
- rubber
- food

Let us now tie in our scientific knowledge to food allergy, hypersensitivity and intolerance.

FOOD HYPERSENSITIVITY

Food hypersensitivity describes an abnormal reaction to food. There are two types of food hypersensitivity:

- **food allergy**

- **food intolerance**

What is the difference between the two? Well one involves the immune system, and the other does not.

FOOD ALLERGY

Food allergy occurs when the immune system inappropriately reacts to a specific food. The food is not really the allergen but rather the specific protein in the food that triggers the immune system. That allergen must come into contact with the person, usually through ingestion. In immediate reactions, the lining of the mouth and throat reacts as the immune system is attacking the allergen as it comes in contact with the lining. The reaction can also be delayed and so there are two main types of a food allergy reactions: immediate (IgE mediated) and delayed (non-IgE mediated).

IMMEDIATE REACTIONS

An immediate reaction happens straight away and up to two hours after eating or coming into contact with the allergen. This immediate reaction is driven by those IgE antibodies I mentioned at the start of this chapter, and you may come across the term 'IgE-mediated' reaction. The release of histamine and other chemicals causes the symptoms and signs which may include:

- itchy mouth

- skin reactions including hives, an itchy rash

- swelling of the face, mouth and/or throat

- difficulty swallowing

- wheezing and difficulty breathing

- low blood pressure

- nausea and vomiting

- hay fever like symptoms, such as sneezing or itchy eyes

- in extreme cases, anaphylaxis (see below) can occur

Note that this is not a complete list of symptoms.

DELAYED REACTION

A delayed reaction takes place between two and 72 hours after ingesting the allergen and is known as a 'non-IgE-mediated' reaction as it is driven by antibodies other than IgE. The main symptoms are:

- itchiness and discoloured skin

- very dry and cracked skin

- vomiting with or without diarrhoea

- indigestion

- constipation

- abdominal cramps

- bloating

- excessive and inconsolable crying

You can see that the symptoms typically involve the skin and bowel. Another distinction between an immediate and a delayed reaction is that with the latter, the child has chronic persistent symptoms really because it is difficult to diagnose leading to continuous exposure to the offending food. The most common cause of delayed reaction is cow's milk allergy. Other causes include soya, egg and wheat allergy. The biggest problem with delayed allergies is diagnosis.

ANAPHYLAXIS

In severe cases of allergy, anaphylaxis can occur. This is a medical emergency and without quick treatment, is life-threatening. The symptoms are sudden and can deteriorate quickly. The initial typical symptoms are those of an immediate reaction followed by:

- a swollen tongue

- difficulty breathing

- tight chest

- trouble swallowing and/or speaking

- dizziness

- collapse

When an anaphylactic reaction occurs, the emergency services must be called immediately to administer immediate treatment. A handy poster guide on symptoms of food allergy with information on anaphylaxis can be downloaded from www.tots2teensallergies.com/thrive

FOOD INTOLERANCE

On the other hand, a food intolerance does not involve the immune system and the symptoms are much less severe than that of a food allergy. Food intolerance can manifest hours or even days after the food has been eaten. One which is very common is lactose intolerance. This happens when an individual does not produce enough *enzymes* to digest the protein in milk. Lactose intolerance is often misdiagnosed as a milk allergy which it is not.

WHICH ONE IS IT?

It is not always easy to determine what is an allergy or intolerance. Let me refer to a quote by Dr Stukus, a leading expert in immunology and paediatric *allergist* at the Food Allergy Centre, Nationwide Children's Hospital, Columbus, Ohio, USA:

'When someone is diagnosed with a new food allergy, it is extremely important for them to receive evidence-based information to guide management at the time they are diagnosed.'

His message highlights three important things:

• there are several steps required to understand if a child has a food allergy or intolerance and how to manage it

• professional help is required – there are quite a few of these steps to diagnosis and management and you should not expect to master these steps alone, and,

• working with healthcare professionals to equip you with the skills to help your child thrive despite their allergies is essential

TYPES OF FOOD ALLERGY

The most common food allergies are to:

- Cow's milk protein
- Egg
- Peanut
- Tree nut
- Fish
- Soya
- Wheat
- Sesame
- Shellfish

COW'S MILK PROTEIN ALLERGY

CMPA is an allergy to one or more protein(s) in cow's milk, usually occurs by the age of six months and is rare after 12 months old. In most cases, a child can outgrow their milk allergy, but in some, CMPA is severe and can result in anaphylaxis. A recent publication in the British Medical Journal (BMJ) in 2021 by Conrado *et al* exploring the national data between 1998 and 2018 showed that in the UK, CMPA was the most common single cause of fatal anaphylaxis[19]. The case of Brooklyn Secor, a nine-year-old girl in Ontario, Canada, highlights this. In 2021, she became the first known case of a child to die because of an anaphylactic reaction to CMPA during a dairy *desensitisation* program (more on desensitisation later). Her mother, Christina Secor, now raises awareness of the importance of having all appropriate precautions in place and remaining vigilant throughout such programmes.

To give a child a good shot at overcoming CMPA, an appropriate management plan guided by a GP and a paediatric dietitian is required. In my daughter's case, we were able to incorporate a *reintroduction* plan. This is the gradual introduction, under guidance, of the allergen to the child's diet in small amounts so that the body can tolerate the allergen. We were committed to it so that by two-and-a-half years old, she had completed reintroduction to both cow's milk and egg. That said every child is different and for some the process takes a lot longer. More on reintroduction and other related terms later.

EGG ALLERGY

This is an allergy to egg proteins. The two proteins that most are allergic to are *ovalbumin* and *ovomucoid*. One significant risk factor for egg allergy is eczema, meaning that those with eczema have a higher chance of also having an allergy to egg protein (see Chapter 2). Other research has suggested that the use of antibiotics in the early years increases the chances of egg allergy. However, this is not certain.

Children who develop an egg allergy often have other allergies to house mites and pollens leading to hay fever. Research has also shown that children who had egg allergy as infants have a significant chance of developing peanut allergy.

A concern many parents of children with egg allergy is whether their child can have a vaccine. This is a legitimate concern as most vaccines have some egg protein (usually ovalbumin). Research has shown that having an egg allergy does not mean they cannot be given the measles, mumps and rubella (*MMR*) vaccine. MMR vaccine is not cultured from hen's egg but in chick embryo fibroblast cell culture. As such it does not contain hen egg allergens in meaningful amounts. *Influenza* and *yellow fever* vaccines do contain egg protein but children with egg allergy can be safely immunized with them in primary care. However, for the influenza vaccine, specialist supervision is required for those who have experienced anaphylaxis to egg[20]. This is also a concern that I have heard from parents of all cultural backgrounds. Remember that vaccines are important and a crucial intervention to help give children the best start in life[21]. They have been shown over the years to be the most effective way to prevent infectious diseases. More recently, we have seen how important vaccination was in controlling the COVID-19 pandemic. If you have concerns about whether your child with an egg allergy can be vaccinated, a conversation with your doctor usually clears things up. The Department of Health – Health Protection in Education and Childcare Settings (Chapter 5) also gives advice on immunization.

PEANUT ALLERGY

Peanut allergy is another food allergy common in children. It usually starts in the first five years of life and is one of the allergies with a huge risk of anaphylaxis. Once a peanut allergy has been diagnosed, strict avoidance is the first step in management. Next is consideration of a prescription for an adrenaline autoinjector then follow up with an allergist to discuss oral *immunotherapy* (OIT), if appropriate. OIT refers to feeding the individual with increasing amounts of the allergen with the aim of increasing the threshold that triggers a reaction. More on OIT later.

There is a misconception that babies and toddlers should not be given peanuts. For babies, the real reason not to do this is to prevent choking. However, peanuts and peanut products may be introduced safely when weaning starts. In a study called the Learning Early About Peanut Allergy (LEAP) study, it was shown that introducing peanuts early was the most effective way to reduce the risk of developing a peanut allergy. It is important though to ensure your child is fit and well when you first introduce age-appropriate peanut-based foods so as not to cloud the presentation of an allergy.

As mentioned before, eczema is also known to be a significant risk factor for developing peanut allergy. This may relate to the impaired skin barrier which is the case with eczema. There is a protein called *filaggrin* which plays a role in the formation of the skin barrier; filaggrin is abnormal in eczema and may also increase the risk of peanut allergy.

A child with peanut allergy is not automatically allergic to other nuts or food items with nut in the name, including coconut or nutmeg. Unfortunately, some parents end up omitting a lot of healthy and tasty nut-based foods for their children which is not ideal for unconfirmed allergies. Avoiding food items that a child is not allergic to deprives them of nutrients and the joy of a varied diet... and creates a fussy eater. It also increases the chances of being allergic to other food items as well.

TREE NUT ALLERGY

Tree nuts include Brazil nuts, hazel nuts, pecans, pistachios, chestnuts, macadamia nuts, cashew nuts, hickory nuts, walnuts, pine nuts and almonds. Tree nut allergy is different from peanut allergy and an allergy to one type of tree nut does not automatically mean an allergy to another. However, both peanut and tree nut allergy can coexist, and a child can have an allergy to one or several tree nuts.

With all allergies, young children may not be able to describe what they are feeling and often spitting out food in distress may be the only sign. It is therefore important to observe a child with new foods and especially if you suspect there is an allergy. This is also why a detailed clinical history is important before testing to confirm the diagnosis. As with peanut allergy, avoiding foods containing the tree nut(s) that lead to an allergic reaction is key.

FISH ALLERGY

Symptoms of an allergy to fish may occur not only after eating it but also just by inhaling the fish vapours during cooking, at the fish counter or market or by skin contact. It is therefore important to be aware of the risk of cross contamination.

The most common type of reaction is an immediate one with the typical symptoms described earlier. Anaphylaxis can also occur. Two important points are:

- Some children with fish allergy can still eat shellfish

- Fish allergy should not be confused with *scombroid poisoning* which is food poisoning that happens after eating fish that has 'gone off'

With fish allergy, it is important to consult an allergist for advice if all fish or just specific ones should be avoided.

SOYA ALLERGY

Soya is a product of soya beans and soya allergy normally starts in infancy. The allergen is the soya proteins. Soya bean is a member of the legume family which also includes beans, peas, lentils and peanuts. Statistics show that 50-60% of babies with delayed CMPA reaction may react to soya as well and will present with gut-related symptoms. On the other hand,

10% of babies with immediate allergic reactions to CMPA react to the soya protein. Most children do outgrow it though some may not. According to FARE, it is rare for those with a peanut allergy to react to soya, but the reverse is not true for those with an allergy to soya.

WHEAT ALLERGY

In Europe, statistics show that about 0.3% of children under the age of 5 have an allergy to wheat[22]. Globally, the prevalence of wheat allergy is estimated to be 1%[17]. A US study in 2009 reported that about 65% of children with a wheat allergy outgrow it by the time they are 12 years old[23]. The allergen here is wheat protein and it can cause either an immediate or delayed allergy. Other symptoms can also include tummy pain and worsening of eczema.

Wheat allergy can be confused with *coeliac disease*. In wheat allergy, the body produces antibodies to proteins found in wheat. On the other hand, in *coeliac disease*, *gluten* in wheat causes a different abnormal immune reaction. The gluten causes inflammation and damage of the lining of the small bowel. In wheat allergy lymphocytic inflammation occurs leading to expression of cytokine proteins called *interleukin*[24]. A schematic illustration on the differences between wheat allergy and coeliac disease can be downloaded from www.tots2teensallergies.com/thrive.

One misconception is that delaying a baby's exposure to wheat during weaning will protect them from developing a wheat allergy. There is no scientific evidence to support this.

SESAME

The incidence of sesame allergy is rising dramatically. It is in fact the most prominent in Middle Eastern countries and the third most common in Israel. Although it does not get as much publicity as peanut allergies, the reactions can be just as severe. Some children can outgrow sesame allergy by the age of six, but it may persist into adulthood.

You may have heard of the case of Natasha Ednan-Laperouse who died in 2016 after an anaphylactic reaction to sesame seeds in a sandwich she had bought before boarding a flight at London's Heathrow Airport. She knew she was allergic to sesame but as the packaging had no allergy labelling, she presumed the sandwich was allergen-free. Natasha's Law, that came into effect in the UK in 2021, is a direct result of this case. It states that pre-packed foods for direct sale must be labelled with a full list of ingredients and allergens. This law protects those with food allergies who rely on transparency of this labelling.

SHELLFISH ALLERGY

Shellfish includes shrimp, prawn, lobster, crab, clam, mussel and oyster. Shellfish allergy is more common in adults than children but is still an important cause of food-induced anaphylaxis in children. Most children with shellfish allergy also have sensitivity to dust mite and cockroach allergens. This is because the allergen in shellfish allergy called *tropomyosin* is also found in house dust mites and cockroaches[25].

There are some other peculiarities to shellfish allergy. First, it is not the same as fish allergy. Children who are allergic to shellfish are usually *not* allergic to white fish, tuna and salmon. However, if a child has an allergy to one type of shellfish, they will generally be allergic to the other types though they may be able to eat molluscs. In some cases, they may also be allergic to fish. As with a fish allergy, symptoms can occur after eating, through inhaling the vapours or via skin contact.

DIAGNOSING FOOD ALLERGY

The diagnosis of any food allergy starts with taking a thorough clinical history of a typical reaction after contact with the allergen. There are a lot of commercial testing panels available, and parents can have allergy tests at a variety of labs. However, many of these labs are not certified to do so and usually there is no one to do that all important first step - taking a thorough history. Only a qualified healthcare professional can do this to make a proper diagnosis of an allergy. More on this in Chapter 4.

Though I have listed the different food allergies separately, I am sure you can understand why it might be difficult to diagnose. For one, our food options are so varied with multiple ingredients in any one food so to identify the allergen will take a lot of effort. The symptoms that children may experience may not be typical ones either. However, I hope I have given you enough of a foundation to build on.

...FINALLY, A WORD OR TWO ABOUT POLLEN FOOD SYNDROME

I must throw some light on this topic for a couple of reasons. Although *pollen food syndrome* (PFS) is a *secondary* allergy that mostly affects adults, children and teens can be affected too. A secondary allergy is one that occurs due to *cross-reactivity*. Cross-reactivity is when the body's immune system identifies the protein in one substance and that in another substance as similar. Secondly, it can be confused with hay fever.

PFS, also known as oral allergy syndrome, is a combination of symptoms and signs that occur when the immune system is triggered by proteins in pollen from trees, grass, weeds and plants. Fruits, vegetables or nuts that have cross-reactivity with pollen in those with hay fever are the usual culprits. The symptoms are usually mild, isolated to the throat and resemble hay fever – runny nose, sore throat, congestion and watery eyes. Anaphylaxis is uncommon but can occur.

For a simple schematic on PFS please check out the resource at www.tots2teensallergies.com/thrive.

Take Home Messages

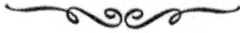

- There are two types of food hypersensitivity: food allergy and food intolerance.

- Food allergy involves the immune system, but food intolerance does not.

- An allergic reaction to an allergen in a food may be immediate or delayed.

- It is important to have a good understanding of food allergy as it is the only way to thrive allergy free.

- The diagnosis of any food allergy and the management plan must be made by an allergist or appropriate healthcare professional (including your GP if they are trained to and a paediatric dietitian with experience on allergy).

Chapter Four

GETTING IT RIGHT

> *"Although disclosing your food allergies in front of others while dining out can be awkward, you can never lose sight of the fact that it is essential. This is one of the most important food allergy management tools, right after avoidance and carrying my auto-injector."* – Hannah Lank, Allergic Living Contributor

The key to thrive free of the limitations that come with having an allergy, or to overcome an allergy, is to get it right – right from the start. This means working with and cooperating with a healthcare professional along what is called a care pathway. This pathway starts with recognising that there might be an allergy then getting specialist input; the specialist then takes a full medical history and fully examines the body before performing allergy testing. After this, a diagnosis can be made which is then followed by putting a management plan in place.

RECOGNISING AN ALLERGY

I shared with you that we eventually suspected that Chimamanda's skin was reacting to something; we could not work out what that 'something' was since I was predominantly breastfeeding; I had only introduced formula milk when she was about three months old because she wasn't putting on weight. So, I could not work out what the possible triggers were. This was the recognition stage for us. When we and our GP had run out of ideas and especially as she had developed a skin infection, we were referred to a paediatric dermatologist.

Today, the NHS has ensured that most GP practices have teams that can recognise and appropriately manage allergies in children and that include a paediatric dietitian. The paediatric dietitian can also diagnose and give treatment. In addition, there is work to make allergy clinics accessible in most GP practices.

It is after this recognition stage that many parents get it wrong. In some cases, a parent sees their child react to a food then, without being clear on whether it is an allergy or intolerance, they exclude that food from the diet. There is no follow up with a GP or dietitian to complete that care pathway. Initial avoidance of the food whether for allergy or intolerance is a good start but the right management plan is required. Here is an example. One day, Nnamdi and I were having a casual chat and he told me about a patient of his, who was perhaps in his mid-50s who did not eat bananas. When my husband probed, the patient went on to say that his mother had told him not to eat bananas and he never did. He never found out why; he just did not eat them. Yes, the old message of managing allergy was to 'avoid, avoid, avoid', but I hope that after reading this book, if you did not already know, there are other routes.

Some parents may go on to get an allergy test themselves without appropriate guidance– whether it is a *food panel test*, *skin prick* or full blood test. This is not generally recommended for a few reasons. The tests can give a *false positive* result, which means that the result may indicate that an allergy is present when it really is not. Without the context of a full history and an examination, or without a follow up management plan, the results are not helpful. A food may then be unnecessarily avoided as a result meaning the child could lose out on vital nutrients or even go on to develop an allergy to that food.

Allergy tests do play an important role in diagnosing IgE-mediated food allergy but require expert interpretation from an allergist or appropriate healthcare professional before making any conclusions. This is what getting it right means. Though it is great that they are available, they are not readily interpretable and so not always useful. It can be said that the increase in these test panels has led to overuse and unnecessary avoidance of many foods.

So, in summary, testing is **not** the first step. If you recognise one of the following:

- your child has one or more of the possible food allergy signs and symptoms, or,

- your child has had treatment for atopic eczema, indigestion or ongoing bowel symptoms that do not respond to simple changes,

then consult with your GP who will work with a paediatric dietitian who is experienced in diagnosing, managing and treating food allergy. In some severe cases or difficult to diagnose cases, an allergist will be involved.

HISTORY AND EXAMINATION

These two steps can only be properly carried out by a specialist. At our first appointment at the dermatology clinic, the specialist nurse took a thorough history and performed a full examination which she discussed with the consultant dermatologist **before** any tests were done.

Current guidance suggests that a history is the most valid 'test'. What is the history? Essentially, this is your child's story. It is taken in detail and provides context.

The history includes asking things like:

- whether allergies run in the family
- what kind of symptoms your child has
- how long the symptoms last
- what foods the symptoms are associated with
- if your child has any other medical conditions, e.g., eczema or asthma
- what your child's quality of life is - how are their activities and interactions affected
- what treatments have already been given

Here are some of the signs the specialist will look for during a physical examination:

- appropriate growth for age
- skin changes
- nutritional state
- other allergy-related conditions, e.g., asthma, eczema

The discussion that takes place after the history and examination is a crucial part of diagnosing and managing any allergy. One thing to note is that the diagnosis is not done and dusted in one step. You may be asked to start a food diary to really pinpoint the trigger. The diary keeps a record of what you observe and should contain:

- what the symptoms of the suspected allergy are, e.g., rash around mouth, itching

- what food was eaten before the symptoms started

- how quickly the symptoms come and disappear

- what you did to soothe the symptoms

So, for example, if putting the history and information from the diary together suggests that the symptoms are mostly delayed, the suspected allergen is excluded for two to six weeks (in most cases, two to four weeks). It is then reintroduced when any symptoms have cleared. The diary should be maintained during the exclusion period and, of course when the suspected allergen is reintroduced. A blank food diary can be downloaded from www.tots2teensallergies.com/thrive

DIAGNOSIS

After the history and examination, and depending on the suspected allergy, your child may be referred to another specialist such as an allergist, paediatric dietitian, or paediatric dermatologist. Any of these specialists may re-examine your child and will choose tests to help in the diagnosis. These may include:

- an elimination diet followed by a planned *rechallenge* or reintroduction

- skin prick tests and specific IgE antibody testing

• sending your child for specialist care

In cases of delayed allergy or non-IgE mediated food allergy, the process is slightly different. The allergen is excluded, then confirmed with a rechallenge and then subsequent reintroduction.

In Chimamanda's case, an IgE antibody test was performed, and the results were available within a few days. The test was positive for CMPA and egg allergy which meant she was reacting to the milk and egg protein in my diet. We were referred to a paediatric dietitian, but in the meantime, I had to stop eating food containing egg and cow's milk if I was to continue breastfeeding. Alongside that, Chimamanda could only drink hypoallergenic milk formula. The first brand prescribed smelt awful and she did not take to it all. We asked for an alternative and our GP prescribed Aptamil® which worked best for her in combination with breast milk. We were also given a plan to manage her severe eczema. This included:

• Oilatum® bath additive

• Zerobase® emollient cream for washing

• Eumovate® ointment to use on the severely affected parts once a day

• Hydrocortisone ointment to use twice a day

• Diprobase® ointment and full body wet wraps

With my background in pharmacology, I was worried about the topical steroids (the hydrocortisone) and their side effects such as skin thinning, but discussions with the specialists cleared my concerns. The history showed that we had tried different creams; however, an ointment was more likely to work best, so here is another reason why that history is important. However, Chimamanda's skin did become fairer with the steroid cream but when we stopped using it, her skin returned to its normal colour over time. For a useful guide on how to choose the appropriate emollient, check out the resource highlighted in Chapter 3 which is available at www.tots2teensallergies.com/thrive

I was not prepared to worry about food allergies at all, especially at Christmas, and specifically, not being able to eat anything with cow's milk and egg. In my research for this book, I found out that medical opinions on the latter differed. Nevertheless, I followed the advice I was given especially because I wanted to continue breastfeeding. I had to embrace it as difficult as it was.

Giving up eggs was easy as I was never a huge fan of them anyway. However, for breakfast, I was a 'cereal-and-cold-milk' kind of girl. So, the thought of not having milk did not go down well. I also love to bake, and eggs, butter, cream and milk are essential. Basically, without them, there was no cake. How on earth was I going to deal with that? For me it was like putting a child in a room full of candy and telling them not to eat any. It was fortunate in a way that the second COVID-19 lockdown of 2020 meant that Christmas was just the three of us, so catering would be much less complicated and less stressful. On Christmas Eve, we made a mad dash to the shops for non-dairy alternatives. I remember spending ages going through ingredient lists - pasta had to be egg-free and it felt like milk protein and egg was everywhere. Was this how life was going to be? I am still not sure how to describe my first egg and cow's milk-free Christmas but all I know was Nnamdi had no idea what it meant as he carried on eating everything as usual!

That year, 2020, was a big year for us with all the changes that came. It started with Chimamanda's appointment with a paediatric dietitian. The first thing I asked was if she would be able to eat eggs and drink milk again, especially as I had read that some children could outgrow CMPA. In addition, I was aware of a project that a former colleague of mine was working on that tested introducing peanuts in small amounts to peanut allergy sufferers. Thankfully, the dietitian told me about the milk and egg *reintroduction ladder* that she was going to use to get my daughter on to cow's milk and egg when it was the right time. More on that later.

THE MEDICAL TEAM

I am sure you have picked up that a variety of healthcare professionals are involved in getting it right. Let me summarise who some of these are:

- **GP** – your local family doctor and your first point of call with any health concerns. They must follow specific steps before referring to a specialist.

- **HEALTH VISITOR** – the person you see often following the birth of your child, either at home or at a community centre. They are very knowledgeable about the needs after childbirth.

- **PAEDIATRICIAN** - a specialist doctor focused on health in children. A general paediatrician is the first point of referral from the GP if a child's medical situation cannot be managed at the general practice.

- **PAEDIATRIC ALLERGIST** – is a doctor who specialises in allergies in children.

- **DERMATOLOGIST** – a doctor who specialises in skin conditions, like eczema.

- **IMMUNOLOGIST** – a doctor who specialises in all aspects of the immune system. They can be involved in the management of an allergy depending on the severity.

- **DIETITIAN** - a healthcare professional whose specialty is in nutrition and diet. In most cases of food allergy, a paediatric dietitian who has a special interest in treating allergies can be involved.

- **SPECIALIST NURSE** – a nurse who has experience and expertise within a specific field of medicine and who works closely with the doctor. They do many of the things doctors used to do. We saw a specialist nurse in paediatric dermatology during our visit to the dermatology clinic and she consulted with the paediatric dermatologist.

- **RESPIRATORY PHYSICIAN** –a specialist in diseases of the lungs. If a child's allergy affects their lungs, they may be involved. Food-induced respiratory reactions can occur which is a component of anaphylaxis. For some children, inhalation of food proteins in the form of aerosols may trigger respiratory symptoms. In cases like this, a respiratory physician may be involved in the management of the food allergy.

Any combination of these specialists can take part in managing a child's allergy, and at any time. It is also important to note that the process might be different in other countries and between public and private care but usually the same professionals are involved.

Take Home Messages

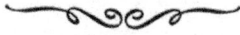

- The first step in diagnosing allergy is getting a clear and complete history of the suspected allergy.

- The first step is **not** an allergy test. Do not use over the counter or online tests yourself but instead be guided by a specialist.

- Getting it right is paramount. It means your child gets the right treatment that does not compromise nutrition and has a chance to recover and thrive allergy free.

- Any combination of specialists may be involved in the diagnosis and management of your child's allergy. It is a process that cannot be rushed.

- For non-IgE mediated food allergies (and some IgE mediated for less severe cases) a management plan can also be made by a paediatric dietitian trained in allergy.

Chapter Five

IT'S NOT A SPRINT, IT'S A MARATHON

> *"Life is a marathon, not a sprint… train for endurance not speed."* – Unknown

After excluding an allergen from a child's diet, it is possible to consider *reintroduction* in a safe environment and only with the guidance of a paediatric dietitian or allergist.

WHAT IS REINTRODUCTION?

Reintroduction is the gradual re-addition of an allergen into a child's diet under medical supervision to train the body's immune system to stop seeing that allergen as foreign. It is a process that must be discussed and jointly agreed on and can take place at home or in the hospital. If there are major concerns about the risk of a severe reaction or anaphylaxis, then your child would be brought into hospital, usually an outpatient clinic, for supervision. Reintroduction is also called 'working up the food ladder' by a lot of paediatric dietitians. Sometimes you may also hear reintroduction referred to as *desensitisation*.

There are two other terms that I will briefly mention. These are *avoidance* and *challenge*. Avoidance is the total exclusion of a food allergen from the diet. In the past, total avoidance was commonly recommended for allergies, but today it is not always necessary. It all depends on the severity of the allergy, the management plan and to what extent the child's body can accept the offending food. It is important that you do not practice avoidance unless it is recommended in your child's management plan. A challenge is performed when a child is introduced to the food that they may be allergic to, to confirm a true allergy.

WHY REINTRODUCTION?

Not all food allergies are for life. Some children may outgrow their allergies as their immune system matures and develops. This is particularly true for CMPA, egg, soya and wheat allergies. On the other hand, some children may not, and this is where re-introduction comes in. Reintroduction is considered a safe way to resume a food considered an allergen to a child's diet. The beauty of reintroduction is that it is monitored, and safety is of paramount importance throughout the process.

Some children with the allergies mentioned above may be able to eat some baked foods such as biscuits (which contain milk) and cake (which contains egg). If they can, you can discuss continuing with these as it can help them outgrow the allergies faster. The tricky thing is that there is no sure way of knowing if a child will outgrow their food allergy. Other allergies such as those to peanut, tree nut, fish and shellfish cannot be outgrown. In such cases, desensitisation through reintroduction and OIT are options when discussing with an allergist. For peanut allergy, an oral drug called Palforzia® is available for children and can help reduce the severity of allergic reactions, including anaphylaxis, that may occur with accidental exposure to peanut. As a scientist working in drug development, it is always a joy to see life-changing treatments move from the lab to real life.

Reintroduction depends on getting the diagnosis right. Let me say from the outset that though it may seem regimented, this can be a time to learn more about your child and to bond. You will be focused on him or her, they on you, and you can, like we did, make it fun, exciting and something to look forward to. It is important to make food enjoyable for children anyway but more so for a child with allergies.

"Never start reintroduction when your child is unwell, even if a mild illness."

REINTRODUCTION – HOW DOES IT WORK?

The key to successful reintroduction is in doing it right to get it right. In this section, I will share how we did it with Chimamanda to illustrate the process. First thing to point out was that we did this in close partnership with the paediatric dietitian. You will remember that soon after Chimamanda was diagnosed, I asked whether she would ever be able to tolerate cow's milk and eggs again. So, this was a goal that was set from the beginning. You can do the same, but it is important to get the expert's opinion on this first before embarking on the journey. Once we started weaning, I was eager to get things rolling with the hope that she would be all set for her first birthday in September 2020. Being the keen baker that I am, my plan was that Chimamanda would have a smash cake and another three-tiered cake for her first birthday photoshoot. That was our second goal and prize at the end of the journey.

FIRST… REINTRODUCTION TO MILK

After our first few meetings with the paediatric dietitian, we agreed to start with milk reintroduction. We used the International Milk Allergy in Primary Care (iMAP) *milk ladder*, and you can download it, as well as some recipes, here www.tots2teensallergies/thrive. The iMAP milk ladder is part of the iMAP Guide, published in 2017 as an evidence-based practical guide for doctors in the UK. It details all the steps from initial presentation, through diagnosis, management and developing tolerance[26]. The ladder gives a stepwise, six-stage guide to reintroducing cow's milk to people with CMPA. I was expecting that we would move smoothly from one level to the next, but things did not fully go to plan.

The first stage, the cookie/biscuit stage, was a breeze. Chimamanda loved the variety of flavours I made. Using grated fruits and puree was a life saver, as at the time, I did not want to introduce sugar to her diet yet. The process was easy for me as a baker. If you are going through this journey with a much older child, it might be a different experience, but the idea is to keep it light and fun.

She passed this stage with flying colours, so we moved on to stage two, the muffin stage. We gave her both savoury and sweet muffins sweetened or flavoured with fruits and vegetables. Again, she sailed through this, so we moved smoothly to stage three, the pancake stage. This one, she did not like one bit, and all this time, I had thought that pancakes were a winner with children. We figured that she just did not 'get' the texture of pancakes, so we had to play around a little with that. After some conversations with the paediatric dietitian, we tried mashed potatoes as an alternative, something she was already comfortable with. Then, I tried mini-pancakes (sometimes called pancake cereal) and served them with different toppings. It was all down to experimenting with textures, which was a challenge, but we persevered, and she eventually moved to the next stage, stage four. This was the cheese stage, and it went by smoothly.

At stage five, the yoghurt stage, Chimamanda reacted with a severe rash. The paediatric dietitian advised us to stop here, allow her skin to clear, then resume the last stage that was not associated with a reaction. For Chimamanda, this meant a month's break then resuming at stage four.

After the second round of stage four was complete, we tried stage five again. This time we spent longer here. This is when I finally realised that the process was not going to be a sprint to the finish line, but rather a marathon. We were in it for the long haul and because it could easily turn into a fraught process, I changed my perception and approach. For this to work with a child, it had to become a real adventure and a time of discovery for each of us in the family. Without this change in approach, it probably would have lasted even longer.

As it turned out, by the time she was a year old in September 2020, she was yet to finish milk reintroduction, let alone start the reintroduction to egg. I had to bake an egg- and dairy-free smash cake for the special day. For added measure, her birthday was during the social restrictions, when we could only meet in groups of six. As such she did not have an elaborate birthday. However, it was a perfect day for just the three of us because in the end, nothing mattered more than her health. The smash cake did not quite manifest as I had hoped because she basically gently patted the cake, which was nonetheless ever so sweet. We also had an online photoshoot session in our living room - a first for us with 'Joy at Home Shoot' organised by Bounty. Following that was a trip to Clarks for her first shoe fitting and a new pair of shoes – a gift from a friend. There was a lot of love and cuddles as the whole day was about her playing and us spending time with her.

A process that I thought would take a few weeks, and at most a few months, turned out to be one that lasted nearly 13 months. Another challenge was that our appointments were all online because of the lockdown period so a lot of modifications had to be made to gather the information needed to monitor her progress. For one we had to take and keep pictures of any observations we made.

I share this part of our story to highlight a few things as you embark on reintroduction with your child. First, patience is paramount especially as there is no defined period over which it should last. Allow your child to progress and flow at his or her pace and be cognisant of the fact that success is on your child's terms and the terms of his or her immune system, not on yours. My mind was set on Chimamanda having a 'normal' cake for her first birthday. She and her body had other ideas though and I had to accept that. There was no way I would have put her health at risk for what I felt should be the perfect 1st birthday. However, it is normal as parents to want our children to smash the goals we set for them, but they will do this only when they are ready. That was a very early lesson for me as a parent and more so as a parent to a child with food allergies.

During Chimamanda's reintroduction, we closely monitored her before, during and after meals, and kept a diary and chart to help us track our observations. This is important to be able to recognise and treat anaphylaxis quickly. It also helps with conversations with the healthcare professionals. Each step was taken under strict guidance and with close cooperation with our medical team which is central to the process.

NEXT... REINTRODUCTION TO EGG

By this time, Chimamanda was one-and-a-half years old. Now that we had some experience, this process was much smoother. There was no pressure, so we really had fun with it, taking our time with each stage. The egg ladder is in two stages. Stage one is cooked egg reintroduction whilst stage two is lightly cooked whole egg reintroduction. If a child has been avoiding all products containing egg, it is advisable to start with stage one. However, if a child can tolerate well-cooked egg in food, then it is advisable to start with stage two. We started with stage one.

"Nnamdi likes eggs and found it difficult when he could not share his meals with Chimamanda, especially as in Nigeria, it is typical for parents, and even grandparents, to share their meal with the children or grandchildren as a show of love. He did not like that he could not do the same with Chimamanda. In addition, families often eat together from the same plate and that is something Nnamdi and I experienced in our childhood.

Chimamanda and I ate separately to avoid cross contamination so we could not carry on that tradition either. One morning, whilst Nnamdi was having breakfast of bread with eggs, Chimamanda walked up to him at the table, and he offered her a piece of bread that he thought had not touched the egg. It turned out it had, and we had not even started the egg challenge yet. As the itching started, panic set-in. Thankfully, we had the oral antihistamine Piriton® that we immediately gave her. I share this incident to tell you that there will be unexpected moments but trust what you have learnt and the medical support you have, to guide you through. It also highlights that it is a process that cannot be rushed, with each stage building on to the other."

Based on the experience above, we were super careful with this phase. We kicked off with a one-egg fairy cake and in fact started by rubbing a small amount of the cake on the inner parts of her lips then waited for 30 minutes. She had no symptoms, so we gave her a pea-sized piece. After two days with no symptoms, we gave her twice the amount we had the first time then waited another two days. We repeated the cycle a few more times until she could eat the full cake. She did, so we moved up to a two-egg fairy cake and repeated the cycle. She also tolerated this well and so we continued feeding her regularly with cake containing egg. Later we added dry pasta and biscuits. All in all, we stayed on the cooked egg stage for a while.

We started stage two the same way with scrambled egg this time. After two days of no symptoms, we progressed to a giving her a pea-sized piece to eat.

Two days later, after no symptoms were observed, we doubled the amount and repeated the cycle, at times allowing a week or two between doses. I wanted to be sure that she tolerated this stage well. Of course, I experimented, adding in omelette and boiled eggs. To be honest, she did not really enjoy any of the textures though she did enjoy an omelette with spinach.

"One thing I did was to make a choice to take the journey with my daughter, following her through the different stages and eating as she did. At one point, Nnamdi was the only person in our household eating egg and milk. Eventually though we all came back together on the same dietary page."

At the end of Chimamanda's journey to thriving allergy free, I was glad that we made the decision to reintroduce from the get-go. This gave us focus as well as an openness to do what it took to make it work for her. There was a lot of compromise, patience, and flexibility no doubt, but the constant motivating factor was wanting our daughter to live as full a life as possible, free from the fear of an allergic reaction. Of course, that was not a guarantee but with the support of all the healthcare professionals, we wanted to give it our best shot and thankfully it worked. If it had not worked, I would still have been grateful that I had tried. At least I would know what she was capable of …and that at least would still allow her to live the best life she could. As you would have observed, we reintroduced our child to cow's milk and egg early towards the end of her weaning. For a more focused guide on reintroduction during this stage of development go to www.tots2teensallergies.com/thrive.

"Remember that every child is different. Some children may not be able to get past a certain stage. It is key to give time and try again because it might take a couple of attempts. It is also crucial to work with the paediatric dietitian or allergist through these processes."

Though I have focused on reintroduction to cow's milk and egg as an example, let me point out a few other things. Reintroduction is used mostly for delayed food allergy but can be tweaked for the more severe IgE mediated food allergy, like peanut allergy, depending on the severity and the plan in place for the child. It is worth mentioning that desensitisation programs can also be offered. Immunotherapy is a treatment option that has a long history for treating other allergies to pollen, bee, wasp venom and pet dander. As highlighted before, Palforia® is the first licensed treatment for peanut allergy. It is given as a series of capsules or sachets containing different doses of peanut protein to gradually increase the exposure to peanut. It is prescribed and can only be given by a trained allergist in the clinic with the support of other healthcare professionals.

Other factors must also be considered during reintroduction. In cases where a child has asthma, for example, the asthma needs to be well controlled before starting. A respiratory reaction for a child with asthma undergoing reintroduction may not just be an asthma attack – it could be a part of the allergic reaction, so you can see where the confusion can arise. With all reintroduction or desensitisation programs, it is important that everyone with the child is aware and understands the signs of a reaction and how to treat it.

A NOTE ON DIET AND NUTRITION...

Finally, I would like to touch on diet and nutrition for both mother and child with a food allergy. Although the focus is constantly on avoiding certain foods, it remains important to maintain a nutritious and balanced diet for baby to grow and mother to recover. A dietitian plays a crucial role here and they do more than just advise on what to eat, for what benefit and when. The dietitian's role and support in caring for a family with food allergies is referred to as medical nutritional therapy[22]. This is personalised and includes an assessment of nutritional status followed by nutrition therapy that includes comprehensive avoidance education while ensuring enough nutrients are available through nutrient-rich alternatives, allergen-free feeding and/or dietary supplements. For example, our dietitian recommended alternatives for Chimamanda before reintroduction. She recommended soya milk when I was weaning her, then a version fortified with nutrients required for one- to three-year-olds when she was older. They can also help you plan the best foods to buy and prepare for you, your child and the rest of the family, and are incredibly supportive in cases where a child with food allergy has siblings without.

Take Home Messages

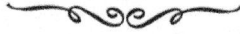

- Reintroduction is not a sprint to recovery but a marathon to victory.

- Close monitoring and professional guidance are essential.

- Be patient. Be open. Be flexible.

- Make reintroduction an adventure for your child.

- Play with textures and flavours as they will not like everything you offer them. I highly recommend using fruits and vegetables as natural sweeteners for children of all ages.

- Whatever the outcome, make reintroduction an opportunity to get to know your child and learn some creative parenting skills.

- Some foods such as nuts may not be suitable for reintroduction. Medical supervision is necessary for managing children with these allergies.

- The role of healthcare professionals cannot be overemphasised in the process of getting it right.

Chapter Six

WHAT ABOUT ME?

> *"Understanding is deeper than knowledge. There are many people who know you, but there are very few people who understand you."* – Nicholas Cage

*I*n this chapter we will focus on you, the parents and carers of a child with food allergy. You are important and need to be taken care of too as this is a journey for the whole family. For those who do not have a child with food allergy, you will get a glimpse of what some parents face and perhaps some ideas on how to best support them.

In the early days of my daughter's allergies, the comments about her became intolerable:

"Tiny, tiny baby."

"She's so tiny."

"She is a tiny baby."

"She is so cute but tiny."

I felt inadequate and insecure especially as a first-time mother who was doing her best to understand this unexpected turn of events. Sometimes I was open about her struggle with food allergy, other times I ignored the comments or avoided situations where these comments could come up.

So, if you are doubting your parental abilities or questioning whether you are doing enough, believe you me when I say, "I get it!" Here is what I focused on to handle these feelings. The first thing to remember is that you cannot control what people say but you can manage how what they say makes you feel. Always remember that you are doing what you can and making the best decisions based on what you know; no one else is walking in your shoes. So don't beat yourself up.

Second, remember that you alone are in charge of how you choose to take the comments of others. Over time, I learnt not to take the various comments as an affront to my abilities as a parent. Instead, I decided these were opportunities to educate others on a family's experience of living with allergies. With that approach, many ended up appreciating what it took to raise a child with food allergy. Pity would turn to admiration and perhaps more consideration when in the company of a 'tiny baby'. Do remain focused on the light at the end of the tunnel; no matter how challenging the journey becomes, there is always going to be another route you can take. Along the way, you are being equipped with what you need to get the result you want.

Let us talk a little more about self-love. As a parent, and especially a mother in those early months when you are the main caregiver, it is natural to focus on caring for your child and forgetting about you (of course it would be the same if the father was the main caregiver). However, I will tell you what my husband would often say to me: "You can't take care of someone if you don't take care of yourself."

I remember going for long periods without taking a break from childcare. That meant extreme fatigue and with that I was easily irritated. I also stopped just taking care of myself; I had always had a healthy head of hair but through neglect, it started breaking. This made me take a step back. Getting the balance right is still a work in progress but now I take care of Uche *and* Chimamanda. Here are my top tips on getting that balance.

PRIORITISE SELF-CARE AND SLEEP

One of the things that I learnt the hard way was how to prioritise self-care. As my mother stayed with us for the first three months of Chimamanda's life, I had been very spoilt. Her staying with us was one of the best gifts my parents gave us especially as I worked right up until I gave birth; I finished work on a Friday and Chimamanda arrived three days later, on the Monday. During those first three months, with mum being around, I had adult conversations when my husband went to work and help around the house. My sleep pattern did not change much, and I could take leisurely showers.

When my mum left, suddenly I had to juggle all these balls that I had no idea existed. At the same time, Chimamanda's allergies were diagnosed. Suddenly, there were days I could not even get round to having a shower or brushing my teeth, and I am someone who used to shower twice a day. Nnamdi, of course, stepped in, helping in the evenings, at night and on his days off. I expressed milk more so that he could support with feeding which is one of the things that makes such a big difference. On one occasion, whilst our daughter napped, he gave me a much-needed back massage. That simple gesture made such a difference.

BE OPTIMISTIC AND KIND TO YOURSELF

I am naturally an optimistic person, so this is perhaps easy for me to say. I remember a work colleague saying to me once, "You always stay positive and calm even when everything around is chaos." Being positive helps a lot especially when in a difficult situation. Even though moments along our journey were very hard, optimism pulled us through.

However, this may not come naturally to you, and you are not alone in this. The good news is that it is possible to retrain your brain to a mode of optimism. To do this, you can start by acknowledging when negative thoughts predominate and specifically counter them with a positive thought or action. It takes practice, like learning any new habit does. Stick with it and you will see it may even rub off on family and friends.

Being optimistic is also about being kind to yourself. The one thing I often told myself was that if I was not nice to me, how could I expect others and life to do the same? The other aspect of this is giving yourself a pat on the back or praising yourself regularly. This shifts the focus from what you think you might have screwed up to what you are winning at, and the bonus is a good dose of positivity.

REMAIN GRATEFUL

The one question I regularly asked myself when it was a struggle was, "Uche, what are you grateful for?" When I felt like a hot mess and that nothing was working, I tried as much as I could to be grateful for what was working. It would go down to the very basic fact that I was grateful to have a child. Yes, the food allergy was a real difficulty, but I was grateful that this was a condition that we could do something about and from which she could recover. I remained grateful for the support system. I was thankful for and celebrated every milestone, no matter what. By the time my daughter's skin had cleared of her eczema, I was well-rehearsed in expressing gratitude.

ACCEPT HELP

It is natural, especially as a new parent, to feel the need to be in control of everything. But you must remember that if you are new at this game, you must learn. To learn, you must be taught and that teaching often comes in the form of help from others. If this is your second- or third time round, having another child adds to your responsibility and every little help someone offers goes a long way. Even with my mother there to help me in the first few months, I still wanted everything done my way. She would always have to remind me to slow down, and I soon realised myself that my approach would not work when it came to living with Chimamanda's allergies.

So, ask for and accept help when it is offered from family, friends, and other support networks. That help may sometimes be a listening ear; I learnt to speak up and share my experiences more and found that this brought me a lot of relief - to talk and to be listened to. Finally, when you do get help, do not forget to enjoy the breaks, guilt-free.

EMBRACE THE FRESH AIR

One of the things that I found therapeutic was going out for walks. Walking cleared my head. The exercise helped me to lose weight and the fresh air helped me mentally. I walked alone, with my daughter in the buggy, with my husband or with friends. The leisurely walks later turned to brisk walks then jogs, boosting my fitness.

After a long walk I could revisit a challenge with a different perspective that allowed me to find a way out of it. The other bonus of walking is that they are a real distraction for your baby. The new sights and sounds open their world and can take their focus away from the anguish that sometimes comes with allergies.

FIND A HOBBY

Having a hobby gives an opportunity to escape from the sometimes-overwhelming demands of parenting a child and especially one with food allergy. It helps with those feelings of inadequacy by reminding you that there is something you enjoy and are good at. My hobby is cake craft, and it was and still is a real escape for me. It takes me to a place where I am creative and free; just modelling chocolate or fondant is relaxing. As it was something I could do at home, it did not require much effort from me.

It is also important to be flexible with our hobbies and little pleasures. I was always the girl with a book to read but I found it impossible when my daughter came into the picture. It would take me ages to finish reading a book if I did finish at all. So, I learnt to listen to audio books and made time to watch a movie or a TV series to compensate.

GET AWAY

Parenting a child with medical needs is demanding and continuous. At times it feels like you cannot step away from it. However, once you feel confident and have trusted family and friends who understand the challenges, stepping back and taking time out is a must. You can start with just 30 minutes away from your child and then gradually build the time up. I remember the first time a dear friend gifted us with her time one evening to take care of our daughter whilst Nnamdi and I went to the movies. This single, simple and free act gave us time to have a date which we had not had for a long time. We talked and laughed and realised how much we had missed being in each other's company; everything we did revolved around our daughter and when that happens it is easy to lose sight of each other. Over time, we have learnt to make a conscious effort to create time just for us. I also got away on my own whilst he took care of Chimamanda.

FORGIVE YOURSELF

Parenting is difficult, period. Then, parenting a child with food allergy or any special needs adds another layer of difficulty. You will sometimes feel, say, or do things you wish you had not. Other times you will feel inadequate when you are unable to alleviate your child's pain. For these moments, forgive yourself. This is important for your parent-child relationship because the unchecked guilt can lead to compensatory behaviour in parenting like impatience and overcompensation.

Take Home Messages

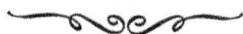

- It is essential to look after yourself as a parent, but especially as a parent of a child with food allergy.

- The ways to do this include prioritising self-care and sleep, being optimistic and kind to yourself, remaining grateful, accepting support, embracing the fresh air, finding a hobby, getting away and forgiving yourself.

Chapter Seven

WHERE ARE WE NOW?

"A journey does not always go as planned. Sometimes all you need to do is let go, trust the process, and see what happens." – Uche Okorji-Obike

I have shared our journey with Chimamanda through eczema, the diagnosis of CMPA and egg allergy and the steps we took to overcoming her allergies. It was clearly not what we had planned for especially as she was our first child. However, it has been a worthwhile road travelled, because she is well, we have this book, Tots2Teens Allergies and an ongoing passion to educate and equip parents with what they need to navigate their own journeys.

As of this moment, Chimamanda is three. How time flies! She was diagnosed at three months old in 2019; reintroduction started at nine months and the process lasted for 13 months. The milk and egg ladders were done in December 2021.

I am going to be honest here and tell you how relieved I was when it was all over. It did not stop me from worrying about what if something went wrong though. I would still ask myself, "What if the allergies returned?" That meant, for example, that I watched her like a hawk when she ate something with egg. However, I have allowed myself to trust the process and have faith that she will be safe. Today, she is doing well, growing into a wonderful, beautiful girl who knows what she wants.

So much has changed since we started. "Mum, can we have egg?" It is such a joy to hear this. When we cook eggs, she says, with such excitement, "We crack an egg!" She also walks up to the fridge, opens it, and points to the bottle of milk for a cup. These moments are priceless as I am reminded of where we started and where we are now. As she is actively involved in her decisions around food and because we share the fun of cooking, she readily sits to eat. So, it is a win all around. Most of all, it is wonderful to share my love of baking with her. Nnamdi now freely shares his food with her without worry. Another bonus us is that sleep is so much better for all of us. In Chapter 1, I shared how we struggled because she would repeatedly wake up because of her sore skin. Today, she is sleeping well, independently… and so are we!

And speaking of her skin, severe eczema is no longer an issue. Occasionally she gets a dry patch around her right wrist. I will say that I have continued with the soap-free bath routine followed by an ointment, though she is no longer using corticosteroids continuously. There is something I noticed though. In the first quarter of 2022, we spent some time in Nigeria; this was Chimamanda's first visit. When we came back to England, her skin became very dry again, and I had to use a lot of wet wraps in the first few weeks. They did work in the end and her skin was back to normal. As such, I think the change from a very warm to a cold climate may have triggered this, though thankfully not as severe as in the past.

Our daughter is like any other three-year-old – full of life and curious – and is meeting her developmental milestones. At nursery, she fully interacts with her classmates. There is never a dull moment with her and so I can truly say that Chimamanda is thriving allergy free. I hope our story has encouraged and inspired you to take the steps that you need to help the child in your life achieve the same.

Chapter Eight

WHAT NEXT?
ACT TODAY

"Action is the foundational key to all success." – Pablo Picasso

$\mathcal{N}$ow that you know all you do about allergies, how can you use that knowledge. The beauty of knowledge is that when you have it, you can act, right? You can take appropriate steps to get the results you want. With the information you have so far, I will encourage you to start putting things in place to ensure you and the child in your life both win!

For some parents the greatest challenge is leaving their child with any allergy in the care of another and the fear that the person might not know what to do in an emergency. That was certainly the case for me because I was hoping to return to work before Chimamanda was a year old. This was despite knowing that most childcare settings now have processes and resources in place to accommodate allergies. There are a few things you can do to help alleviate these fears.

KEEP AN 'ESSENTIALS BAG' READY

The same approach to having a hospital bag for baby's arrival or a cabin bag ready if you fly often is applied here. If your child is at nursery or school, a bag should also be kept there. What are the essentials in this case?

- **Medication** - antihistamines

- **Adrenaline Auto-Injector** - an automatic injection device designed to deliver a dose of adrenaline to treat anaphylaxis

- **Instructions** on what to do in the event of an allergic reaction

You can create a simple instruction card so that the responsible adult taking care of your child will know what to do in case of an emergency. A sample can be downloaded from www.tots2teensallergies.com/thrive

USE AN IDENTIFIER

An alert bracelet or badge is used to ensure that others are easily able to recognise a child that has a food allergy. Some parents may feel that this will single out their child as different from others, but it is a quick way for caregivers to identify when they need to take extra care.

EDUCATE FAMILY AND FRIENDS

This cannot be over emphasised. It is important for parents of children with food allergy to communicate, communicate and communicate. The aim is to share the burden and ensure your child's safety.

EDUCATE YOUR CHILD

This should be done in a loving and age-appropriate way. Be prepared to repeat a lot, patiently, to be sure they 'get it'. Gently explain to them that everyone is different, and everyone's needs are different. Show them what they can do for themselves which gives them security and confidence. There are also story books and other resources for children with allergies to help communicate the concept. Part of the management plan is to prepare your child for the outside world beyond the shores of your home. You empower your child when you educate them which is essential to help them thrive allergy free.

EDUCATE THE SCHOOL

This also applies to nursery even though they will have their own processes. In fact, ask for the school's procedures and protocols for managing allergies. If there are additional steps required for your child which are not covered, you can highlight this to the teachers. In most cases, a clinical nurse specialist may be invited to educate the staff annually especially as team members change. However, this does not replace an emergency plan or any other specific management plan that your child has been given.

Your child may not like all this 'fuss' as it singles them out as different from others. However, as you continuously educate your child, he or she will get to understand that it is all for their own good.

PLAN TRAVEL

We did not travel much with Chimamanda as she was diagnosed during the COVID19 pandemic. However, when restrictions lifted, we took short breaks within the UK. These are my top tips and must-haves for travel.

1. Consider translation cards for foreign trips. They are handy especially with eating out. Allergy UK has a range of those.

2. An emergency card to highlight the risk of an anaphylactic reaction is important as it communicates the gravity of such a reaction.

3. Your emergency contact details should be easily accessible.

SOCIAL EVENTS

It is important that your hosts know your child's dietary requirements in good time. At times though I still carried food with me just in case. Other things to do are:

1. Consider having an ally who can help keep an eye on your child.

2. Always check the contents of the party bags.

3. Provide instructions on what to do in an emergency.

4. If your child is going to an event alone, educate him or her and inform the organisers on what to do in the event of a reaction.

Take Home Messages

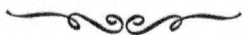

- Act on the knowledge you now have.

- With adequate preparation and education, you can be confident that your child can be safe outside the shores of your home.

- It is important to empower and teach your child on what to do to avoid and treat allergic reactions. This gives them the confidence to thrive allergy free and without fear.

Chapter Nine

FINAL THOUGHTS

"A stitch in time saves nine." – Unknown

I have shared Chimamanda's journey with food allergies and weaved in some insights into the biology behind this rising phenomenon. My hope is that after reading the book, you now have a better understanding of food allergies as well as the challenges one can face. I also hope you have been able to pick up some tools that can help your child or a child around you with food allergies to thrive allergy free.

It can be a challenging road for the whole family but if you adopt some of the principles outlined in this book, some of those challenges can be managed. First, it is important to get professional help; this book does not replace that. I am a scientist, and my husband is a medical doctor, yet even with our combined knowledge, we still needed help – and that was not a bad thing. This was not something we could fix ourselves. Second, as you work towards helping your child to thrive allergy free, do not forget to have some fun. Do not be too hard on yourselves. Take it as at time to learn and grow together. There will be some hard days; allow these to run their course and always remember to bring the focus back to the goal.

The journey can be lonely at times. That is one of the reasons why I created Tots2Teens Allergies - as a place where families and friends dealing with food allergies can be part of a supportive community. I urge you to access this space, explore it, come back to it, and I am sure you will find something, even just one thing, for you. That resource space and this book will set you and your child on the path to thriving allergy free.

GLOSSARY

Acid mantle - a thin film on the skin surface composed of fats from the oil glands mixed with amino acids from sweat

Alkaline - relating to or containing properties of alkaline; the opposite of acidic

Allergen - trigger for an allergy/allergic reaction; under normal circumstances these are normally harmless (see **trigger**)

Allergenic – having the capacity to case an allergic reaction

Allergy - a reaction produced by the immune system when exposed to an allergen

Antibody - a large protein used by the body's immune system to identify and neutralise foreign substances; they help fight infection (see **Immunoglobulin**)

Antihistamine – a drug that blocks the effects of histamine, the substance that causes some of the effects of an allergic reaction like sneezing, itchy eyes and runny nose; can be bought over the counter or prescribed

Atopic dermatitis - an allergic condition that makes the skin discoloured and/or itchy.; common in children; can be long lasting with a tendency to periodic flare ups

Autoimmune disease - an illness that occurs when the immune system cannot tell the difference between the body's own cells and foreign cells, leading to the body mistakenly attacking normal cells

Avoidance – taking measures to remove an allergen from the diet

Blood IgE - refers to the level of IgE protein in the blood (see **Immunoglobulin E**)

Caesarean section – a surgical procedure where a baby is removed from the uterus of the mother by cutting the mother's abdomen

Cell-mediated – the reaction of the immune system that does not involve antibodies but instead cells of the immune system

Challenge – when a food is given gradually in increasing amounts, under medical supervision, to either accurately diagnose or rule out a food allergy

Coeliac disease - a disease in which the small intestine is oversensitive to gluten, making it difficult to digest gluten

Contact dermatitis - a type of eczema triggered by contact with a particular substance

Cradle cap – crusty or oily scales on a baby's scalp; it is harmless, not related to hygiene and usually clears up on its own

Cross-reactivity – when proteins in one substance are like proteins in another substance and so may cause the same reaction

Cytokine – chemicals made by the immune system that either stimulate it or dampen it down

Dermatitis - a general term that describes a skin irritation; has many causes and forms and causes dry, itchy or discoloured skin, or a rash

Dermatology – a speciality in medicine that deals with conditions of the skin

Desensitisation – giving small quantities of an allergen daily to make the immune system become insensitive or used to it

Dyshidrotic eczema - a type of eczema that affects the hands or feet; usually a long-term condition with first symptom often being a burning or prickling feeling in the affected area; also called 'pompholyx'

Eczema - a condition that causes the skin to become itchy, dry and cracked

Enzymes – proteins in the body that speed up our chemical reactions

Filaggrin – a protein that plays an important role in the strength of the skin barrier

Food allergy - a reaction of the immune system which occurs when an individual eats food containing an allergen

Food hypersensitivity - an adverse reaction to food which causes unpleasant symptoms that can be life-threatening; there are two types of food hypersensitivity: food allergy and food intolerance

Food intolerance - difficulty in digesting certain foods resulting in unpleasant reactions; symptoms include tummy pain and bloating

Food panel test – a blood test that measures antibodies to a range of the most commonly eaten foods

Gluten – a protein found in grains like wheat, barley or rye

Gut flora - the collection of bacteria that live in the gut

Histamine – a chemical of the immune system that kickstarts the process of getting rid of a trigger

Hypoallergenic – used to describe something that has a low number of substances that are likely to cause an allergic reaction

iMAP - International Milk Allergy in Primary Care; a guidance used in the management of mild to moderate milk allergy

iMAP milk ladder - a guidance used for reintroduction of cow's milk to the diet

Immune system - a network of cells, organs, proteins known as *antibodies* and chemicals that together function as a safety surveillance system for the body

Immune-mediated response - the response driven by the immune system following a reaction to an allergen

Immunoglobulin E (IgE) - a type of antibody found only in mammals and manifests in allergic diseases (see **Blood IgE**)

Immunoglobulin - another name for antibodies

Immunotherapy - a type of treatment that influences or modulates the immune system so that it does what it should do

Inflammation – the process that takes place when the immune system responds to a harmful substance, infection, injury or trigger; the hallmarks of inflammation are redness, heat/warmth, swelling, pain and loss of normal function

Influenza - a contagious illness that infects the nose, throat and sometimes lungs

Interleukin – proteins made by the white blood cells of the immune system that usually stimulate the immune system

Microbes - organisms that are small and only seen under a microscope; include bacteria, fungi and viruses

MMR vaccine - the measles, mumps and rubella vaccine; a safe and effective combined vaccine

Neonatal - a new-born or a child in the first 28 days of life

Oral immunotherapy - where small quantities of a food allergen are eaten every day under supervision to gradually building the body's resistance to that allergen

Ovalbumin – the main protein found in egg white

Ovomucoid – another protein found in egg white but in lesser quantities than ovalbumin

Pollen food syndrome – a condition where the individual is allergic to pollen, raw fruits, vegetables and some tree nuts; there is cross-reactivity to the proteins in these foods (see **secondary allergy**)

pH - an expression of how acidic or alkaline a solution is

Prebiotics – foods that promote the growth of good bacteria in the gut (bacteria feed on these foods); these foods are usually a type of fibre

Probiotics - 'good', 'friendly' and live bacteria and yeasts that help restore the natural balance of bacteria in the gut; usually added to yoghurts or taken as food supplements

Protein - a macronutrient that is essential to building muscle mass

Reintroduction - the gradual re-addition of a food allergen to a person's diet

Reintroduction ladder – a guide used for reintroducing an allergen into the diet of a child with an allergy

Seborrheic dermatitis - a common skin condition that mainly affects the scalp. It causes scaly patches, inflamed skin and stubborn dandruff; can also affect other oily areas of the body like the face, nose, eyebrows, ears, eyelids and chest

Secondary allergy - an allergic reaction that occurs soon after eating raw fruits and/or vegetables; symptoms can include itching and tingling of the lips, mouth and throat and is also known as 'oral allergy syndrome', 'cross-reactivity' or 'pollen-food syndrome'

Skin prick test - a scratch or puncture test of the skin that checks for immediate allergic reactions to known allergens; used to diagnose allergies

Tropomyosin - a protein found in muscle

Trigger - substances that can aggravate the immune system leading to flare ups of eczema and allergies (see **allergen**)

Yellow fever - a disease caused by a virus that is spread through mosquito bites; symptoms include fever, chills, headache, backache and muscle ache

REFERENCES

1. BSACI resources on Allergy (www.bsaci.org)
2. Loh W and Tang MK (2018) The Epidemiology of Food allergy in the Global Context. *Int J Environ Res Public Health.* 15 (9): 2043. doi: 10.3390/ijerph1509243
3. Natasha Allergy Research Foundation (www.narf.org.uk)
4. Perkin MR *et al.* (2016) Randomized Trial of Introduction of Allergenic Foods in Breast-fed Infants. *The New England Journal of Medicine.* 374:1733-1743. doi:10.1056/NEJMoa1514210
5. Martin P.E, Eckert J, Koplin J.J., and Lowe A.J. (2014) Which infants with eczema are at risk of food allergy? Results from a population-based study. *Clinical and Experimental Allergy* 45(1) doi:10.1111/cea.12406
6. Chiu C Y, *et al.* (2019) Early-onset eczema is associated with increased milk sensitization and risk of rhinitis and asthma in early childhood. *Journal of microbiology, immunology, and infection.* 53(6) doi: 10.1016/j.jmii.2019.04.007
7. National Institute for Health and Clinical Excellence (NICE) guidance. Food allergy in children and young people. https://www.nice.org.uk/guidance/cg116/evidence/full-guideline-136470061 (Accessed March 2022)
8. Breastfeeding Network UK: https://www.breastfeedingnetwork.org.uk/cows-milk-protein-allergy-cmpa-and-breastfeeding/#:~:text=Cow's%20milk%20protein%20allergy%20(CMPA)%20can%20affect%20people%20of%20all,0.5%25%20of%20exclusively%20breastfed%20babies. (accessed 21 September 2022)
9. Al-Ahmed et al. (2008) Peanut Allergy: An Overview. *Allergy Asthma and Clinical Immunology* 4(4): 139 – 143. doi:10.1186/1710-1492-4-4-139

10. Kagan RS, *et al.* (2003) Prevalence of peanut allergy in primary-school children in Montreal, Canada. *J Allergy Clin Immunol* 112:1223–8.

11. Peters RL, *et al.* (2017); HealthNuts Study. The prevalence of food allergy and other allergic diseases in early childhood in a population-based study: HealthNuts age 4-year follow-up. *J Allergy Clin Immunol.* 140(1):145-153.e8. doi: 10.1016/j.jaci.2017.02.019. Epub 2017 May 14. PMID: 28514997.

12. Flom JD and Sicherer SH (2019) Epidemiology of Cow's Milk Allergy. *Nutrients.* 11 (5):1051. doi:10.3390/nu11051051, PMID:31083388

13. Caffarelli et al (2010) Cow's milk protein allergy in children: a practical guide. *The Italian journal of paediatrics.* 36(1):5. doi:10.1186/1824-7288-36-5

14. Pensabene L et al. (2018) Cow's Milk Protein Allergy in Infancy: A Risk Factor for functional Gastrointestinal Disorders in Children? *Nutrients.* 10(11):1716. doi: 10.3390/nu10111716.

15. Sancheza J and Sancheza A (2015) Epidemiology of food allergy in Latin America. *Allergologia et Immunopathologia* 43(2) 185-195 doi: 10.1016/j.aller.2013.07.001

16. Kung S-J, Steenhoff AP and Gray C. (2014) Food Allergy in Africa: Myth or Reality? *Clinical Reviews in Allergy & Immunology.* 46, 241–249 doi: 10.1007/s12016-012-8341

17. FARE (https://www.foodallergy.org/resources/facts-and-statistics)

18. Peters RL, *et al.* (2021) Update on food allergy. *Paediatric Allergy and Immunology.* 32 (4):647 – 657. doi: 10.1111/pai.13443

19. Conrado A.B., Ierodiakonou D, Gowland M.H., Boyle R.J., Turner PJ. (2021) Food anaphylaxis in the United Kingdom: analysis of national data, 1998-2018. *British Medical Journal (BMJ).* 372:n251. doi.org/10.1136/bmj.n251

20. Leech S.C., *et al.* (2021) BSACI 2021 guideline for the management of egg allergy. https://doi.org/10.1111/cea.14009.

21. Department of Health – Health protection in education and childcare settings. Chapter 5. https://www.gov.uk/government/publications/health-protection-in-schools-and-other-childcare-facilities/chapter-5-immunisation Date accessed 18th Sept 2022

22. European Centre for Allergy Research Foundation (ECARF) https://www.ecarf.org/en/information-portal/allergies-overview/wheat-allergy/ Date accessed March 2022

23. Keet CA, Matsui EC, Dhillon G, Lenehan P, Paterakis M, Wood RA (2009). The natural history of wheat allergy. *Ann Allergy Asthma Immunology* 102 (5) 410 – 415

24. Cianferoni A. (2016) Wheat allergy: diagnosis and management. *J Asthma Allergy*. (9) 13-25. doi: 10.2147/JAA.S81550

25. Wong L, Huang CH, Lee BW (2016) Shellfish and House Dust Mite Allergies: Is the link Tropomyosin? *Allergy Asthma Immunol Res*. 8(2) 101 – 106 doi: 10.4168/aair.2016.8.2.101

26. Fox A, Brown T, Walsh J, Venter C, Meyer R, Nowak-Wegrzyn, Levin M, Spawls H, Beatson J, Lovis M-T, Vieira MC, Fleischer D. (2019) An update to the Milk Allergy in Primary Care guideline. *Clinical and Translational Allergy* 9(40) doi.org/10.1186/s13601-019-0281-8

27. Groetch ME, Christie L, Vargas PA, Jones SM, Scicherer SH (2010) Food allergy educational needs of pediatric dietitians: a survey by the Consortium of Food allergy Research. *Journal of Nutrition Education and Behaviour*. 42 (4):259-264.doi:10.1016/j.jeb.2009.06.003

ADDITIONAL RESOURCES

These resources have been highlighted throughout the book and are available at www.tots2teensallergies.com/thrive. They are downloadable illustrations that can serve as flashcards, posters or guide materials to support you and your child.

- · 3 Es of Learning
- Recommended skincare routine for eczema
- How to make a wet wrap for eczema
- Types of emollients
- The immune system and allergic reactions
- The types of food hypersensitivity
- Symptoms of allergic reactions
- Triage of anaphylaxis
- Differences between wheat allergy and coeliac disease
- Pollen cross-reactivity chart
- Blank food diary
- Egg ladder for reintroduction
- Milk ladder for reintroduction
- Guide on reintroduction during weaning
- Recipes for reintroduction
- Food allergy essential bag instruction card

https://www.itchysneezywheezy.co.uk/public.html

https://www.rcpch.ac.uk/resources/clinical-guidelines-evidence-reviews/allergy-care-pathways

ABOUT THE AUTHOR

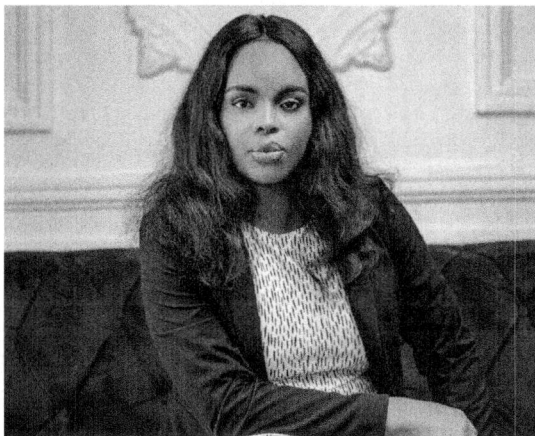

Uche Okorji-Obike, BSc, MSc, PhD, is mother to a gorgeous girl, Chimamanda - the inspiration behind this book and the resource site, Tots2Teens Allergies.

With both, Uche's goal is to help make life 'easy-peasy' for families of children with allergies. The book chronicles her and her husband's journey with Chimamanda and her allergies – the struggles, successes and opportunities.

Chimamanda developed allergies to cow's milk and egg as a baby. As a mother and an expert in inflammation - the subject of her PhD and the underlying mechanism for allergies - Uche's interest in understanding and managing the triggers of Chimamanda's allergies took on a whole new meaning. Along the way, she founded Tots2Teens Allergies which she hopes will become a definitive resource for parents, carers and healthcare professionals looking after their precious little… and big ones with allergies.

Uche has a BSc in Pharmacology from the University of Aberdeen, an MSc in Drug Discovery from the University of Bradford and a PhD in Pharmacology from the University of Huddersfield where her focus was on neuroinflammation. In 2014, she received an award for her work from the Association of Women Graduates (Huddersfield Chapter), a part of the British Federation of Women Graduates. Since completing her PhD, she has been working in the pharmaceutical industry supporting the development of new treatments for various diseases. She is also a member of BSACI - the British Society for Allergy and Clinical Immunology and holds a Nutrition and Wellbeing Certificate (2020) from the University of Aberdeen.

"I hope everyone that picks up this book learns something new that can help them support someone with allergies, be it their own child, a relative, friend, colleague or neighbour."

Printed in Dunstable, United Kingdom